9 Simple Solutions to Achieve HEALTH EQUITY

9 Simple Solutions to Achieve HEALTH EQUITY

A Guide for Healthcare Professionals and Patients

Mauvareen Beverley, MD

Copyright © 2024 by Mauvareen Beverley, MD

All rights reserved.
No portion of this book may be reproduced in any form without written permission from the publisher or author, except as permitted by U.S. copyright law.

ISBN (paperback): 979-8-218-44668-0
ISBN (ebook): 979-8-218-44679-6

Book design and production by www.AuthorSuccess.com

Printed in the United States of America

My book is dedicated to the individual patients of all races, ethnicities, and nationalities who are in our hospital beds and not in the history books . . . those who were instrumental in providing boots-on-the-ground solutions to achieve health equity.

Praise from a patient
"My name is Cassandra Dobson, PhD. I am a patient with Sickle cell disease (SCD). The lack of human value, empathy, caring that Dr. Beverley talks about in her book, is what I experienced when I was hospitalized. I truly believe if the perception vs. the reality of the individual is not correct, poor health outcomes are highly likely. In my case it had nothing to do with social determinants of health as I am an African American Professor and fully insured. I am so thankful that Dr. Beverley intervened on my behalf and as a result I am here today to tell my story as a validation of her book! Please make sure everyone reads her book as it's a game changer for all communities, particularly the AfricanAmerican/Black community."

"It is more important to know the person who has the disease than the disease who has the person."
—Hippocrates

"In Jamaica, I Feel Like A Human Being."
—Dr. Martin Luther King, Jr. (1965)

Contents

Preface		xi
Introduction		1

SECTION I   7

CHAPTER 1:	A Brief History of the Health Crisis of Blacks in the United States	9
CHAPTER 2:	Harlem on My Mind	17
CHAPTER 3:	Queens Health Network: Care Management Program Ahead of its Time	28
CHAPTER 4:	Kings County Hospital—Merging of The African Diaspora	49
CHAPTER 5:	Medications and Adherence	77
CHAPTER 6:	Two Illuminating Patient Stories	84

SECTION II   93

CHAPTER 7:	Nine Simple Solutions for Addressing Health Disparities and Achieving Health Equity	95
CHAPTER 8:	Improving the Patient Engagement and Cultural Competence Experience Training: A Road Map	112
CHAPTER 9:	Six Scenarios for Health Systems and Healthcare Providers to Implement and Address	125
CONCLUSION		128

SECTION III 131

RESOURCES 133
Health Disparities in the United States—Statistics 133
NOTES 140
ACKNOWLEDGMENTS 141

Preface

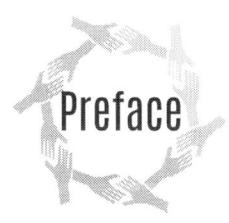

Throughout my professional medical career, I have been fortunate to have worked in various hospitals, and alongside other amazing healthcare professionals who have shaped my values on patient engagement and Care Management. I have had the privilege and humbling experiences of caring for, and learning from patients, caregivers, and families from diverse cultures and social backgrounds in New York City. Achieving the best patient outcomes requires more than practicing good medicine. It also requires an understanding and appreciation of a non-judgmental patient engagement, and a mindset that values the patient as a human being and not as a disease or condition. The unique engagements I had with various staff, those encounters I experienced with patients and their families, and the resulting initiatives I implemented, led me to create this guide. All these experiences have been a major testament to the contents of this book.

Reflecting on my experiences as an intern and resident in the Department of Medicine at Harlem Hospital where excellence in healthcare for *all* patients was the expectation and the norm. Under the leadership of Director of Medicine Dr. Gerald E. Thomson, we all had to provide excellent and quality care to all patients irrespective of race, gender, or employment status. Under Dr. Thomson's leadership, we understood and recognized the mandate to provide excellent care, regardless of circumstances. As one of the public hospitals in New York City, we took care of patients from diverse socioeconomic backgrounds, including severely ill patients with challenging health conditions. There was a relative lack of resources at public health hospitals compared to the well-funded private institutions, such that as interns we also had to transport patients from the emergency department to the inpatient unit and to radiology for needed X-rays for diagnostic purposes and rotate inpatient beds to accommodate admissions in male and female rooms. This was all in addition to our clinical duties. Despite the environment of scarce hospital resources, Dr. Thomson inspired and encouraged us to provide the highest quality care for all patients.

Nine Simple Solutions to Achieve Health Equity describes some of the innovative and unique initiatives I developed for promoting patient-centered quality care, including the first Care Management Program at NYC Health and Hospitals, Queens Health Network (QHN). The cornerstone of this innovative program was to foster better communication and engagement between healthcare clinical teams and patients. An impactful initiative of the Care Management program was the establishment of The Bridge Team. The goal of the Bridge Team was to bridge the gaps in care for the patient population and their families, and in particular, for those that were most vulnerable to adverse experiences and worse health outcomes.

Dr. Thomson was a visionary leader who embedded ideals of "equality," specifically our responsibility as physicians, to treat and value all patients alike, without regard to race, ethnicity, gender, socioeconomic status, physical, mental health, or substance abuse status. I had the opportunity to pose a question to several physicians that trained with me at Harlem Hospital. I asked, "If there were more leaders like Dr. Thomson, in the current roles of chief medical officers (CMO) or chief executive officers (CEO) in our hospitals today, would we be talking about *addressing* health **disparity** or about *achieving* health **equity**?"

All of them responded, "Health equity."

So, what is in this book? This book is my attempt to share boots-on-the-ground simple solutions as well as an outside-the-box innovative approach to moving from tackling health disparities to achieving health equity within healthcare settings. I try to frame a roadmap in stages so that anyone can implement it effectively. I provide stories and examples of scenarios to make them relevant and applicable. I share some of the complex challenges we see within healthcare, resulting from the perception versus the reality of experiences, information, and true perspectives of the population served. The resulting false perceptions and missed communication leads to misunderstanding, contributing to poor health outcomes. I share the need to recognize that there are simple solutions to prevent escalation to the need for complex solutions, if we choose to accept and address them in a non-judgmental, humane, and empathetic manner.

This book is intended to educate all healthcare professionals, practitioners, and patients. It is important to understand that a patient is more than being just an individual with a disease condition. The individual who happens to be a patient may also be a mother, a father, a grandparent, a devoted church member, a minister, or an accomplished teacher in their community.

I also focus on the importance of patient engagement and cultural competence for English-speaking, limited English-speaking, and non-English-speaking populations. Equally important is the fact that the English-speaking Black patient population is not included in the need for cultural competence. It is important to ensure that the doctors, as well as the entire clinical or Care Management team, appreciate patients as individuals, with values and beliefs shaped by their culture or lived experiences.

Finally, I provide some important historical highlights of the health crisis of the Black population. It is unconscionable, when one considers the atrocities that they have endured over the course of history, for the Black American population to continue to experience overall less access to quality care, with worse health outcomes. Whether it be pulmonary, cardiac, urology, infectious disease, kidney disease, or the COVID-19 pandemic—they have the worst health outcomes. We must fix this.

Introduction

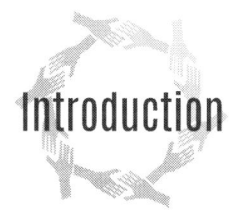

One week while working in the role as Deputy Executive Director of Care and Case Management at King's County Hospital, I was notified about an eighty-two-year-old African American patient who had been admitted with heart failure. After a few days in the hospital, the woman had stopped eating, was not actively participating in her own care, and appeared to be depressed. The clinical team charged with her medical care was baffled by her decline and recommended that she receive a psychiatric evaluation for depression screening.

I agreed that a psych evaluation was warranted but wondered if something more might be affecting the patient's condition. So, that Wednesday I visited her in her hospital room, introduced myself, and asked, "What is important to you? What are you worrying about?"

Expecting her to speak about her medical symptoms, I wasn't surprised when she said, "I am most concerned that I won't be able to get to church on Sunday. It is especially important to me that I please God, and not going to church would make me feel guilty."

Based on that conversation, I had my team contact the woman's minister and arrange a visit from him. He assured her that if she were not discharged from the hospital by Sunday, he himself would come back to pray with her. Once she received that reassurance, she resumed eating, became much more cooperative in her treatment, and appeared much less depressed.

This true story is an example of how health disparities often arise due to lack of cultural competence for care of the elderly Black population, which contributes to a lack of understanding of the individual patient. In this case, it was important for the clinical team to account for the significant role religion played in the patient's life. As is true in most healthcare environments, hospitals do not necessarily have a system in place that recognizes the role of religion in the health and well-being of the Black population, as they do with other populations. The classical Greek physician Hippocrates, who lived from 460 to 370 B.C., once said, "It's more important to know the person who has the disease than the disease who has the person."

Thousands of years ago, he understood this basic medical truth that modern-day healthcare professionals are just now rediscovering.

This book, *Nine Simple Solutions to Achieve Health Equity: A Guide for Healthcare Professionals and Patients*, provides some approaches and solutions to address some of the long-standing health disparities experienced by the Black population in America. Health disparities impact various racial and ethnic population groups to different extents; however, poorer health status and adverse outcomes experienced by the Black population affect all ages, socioeconomic status, and disease categories. If we improve the health outcomes of African Americans, the group that historically experiences the worst health disparities and health outcomes, we can improve healthcare for all populations.

Nine Simple Solutions to Achieve Health Equity promotes health equity by recognizing the human value of *all* patients through the concept of the common thread: the human experience. This common thread, which applies to *everyone*, is the fact that once a disease is accurately diagnosed it is *non-negotiable* and cannot be given back, irrespective of the patient's race, ethnicity, socioeconomic status, gender, religion, or country of origin. In other words, the same applies to a billionaire as well as a homeless individual. The billionaire can't buy his or her way out of an illness by saying, "I will give you a million dollars to take the cancer back. Oh, that's not enough? Then I will give you five million."

Both share the common thread of having a non-negotiable disease. If we accept this concept of our shared common thread—the human experience—then *all* patients will be treated equally with empathy rather than receiving inequitable care based upon discriminatory bias and judgmental attitudes.

To achieve this kind of health equity, we must identify the concerns and needs of our various populations—particularly the elderly Black population—as they have the worst health outcomes in all disease categories. We need to include them in the health equity strategy conversation. For solutions to be viable, they must engage patients, ask questions, and understand their healthcare experiences. This can only be determined by gathering information from patients within the healthcare system.

This book will explain how to foster productive dialogues between doctors and patients to promote health professional *cultural sensitivity and organizational cultural competence*. Cultural sensitivity and organizational cultural competence in this context refer to the ability of providers and organizations to effectively deliver healthcare services that meet the social, cultural, and linguistic needs of patients. Throughout my career, I have dedicated myself to listening to patients and acknowledging the stop-in-your-tracks moments caused by these conversations, which I have recognized to be a new truth about health equity. I have included many of these patients' stories here in this book and based my strategies on the information gained from them.

One thing that makes this book unique is that it presents boots-on-the-ground practical and sustainable solutions for implementation of needed processes in promoting health equity. I will guide you through nine solutions and explain how to apply them in various healthcare scenarios. There are valuable communication tools presented, such as the *Spot Check Methodology, CHANGE Pneumonic* and the *Why? Tool*, used to address the overuse of the label "noncompliant."

Nine Simple Solutions to Achieve Health Equity is especially helpful to physicians because it highlights valuable information on how to improve patient engagement through cultural sensitivity by providing the tools needed to recognize the individual human value of the patient rather than judging, based on a conscious or unconscious bias. This allows for unbiased and quality patient care without regard to race or ethnicity. I discuss the need for unique cultural sensitivity training between American-born physicians with foreign-born patients, foreign-born physicians with American-born patients, and American-born physicians with American-born patients who are different from themselves. All patients are part of the shared human experience.

This book is also meant to be a valuable resource for patients because it provides essential information and tools to improve interaction and dialogue with doctors, nurses, and social workers, by first and foremost communicating who you are as an individual, your fears, what's important to you, and where you are in the acceptance of your disease. This is vital information for you to provide, so that you receive the person-centered health and equitable care you deserve.

This book is divided into three sections.

Section I begins with a discussion of the current conditions of health disparity in the United States, especially as experienced by the Black population. I present a brief history of the problem, and how it got to be the way it is today. After that, I discuss my experiences at various hospitals and how they shaped my professional opinions about health equity and inspired me to develop the concepts mentioned in this book.

In **Section II**, I describe the **nine simple solutions** to achieve health equity, beginning with an overview of the concepts followed by a look at how these ideas are particularly relevant to health professionals and the patient-caregiver community. I subsequently examine some case studies of these strategies in action.

Finally, in **Section III**, I provide additional information and identify a few resources that you may find to be helpful in your own journey toward health equity.

Achieving health equity for all populations, especially the Black population, is necessary and doable. I am humbled to propose some easy-to-implement solutions based on my experiences, and information shared directly from patients. I present these innovative processes so they may be utilized by clinical teams including physicians, physician assistants, nurses, social workers, and patients. Let's get started.

SECTION I

CHAPTER 1

A Brief History of the Health Crisis of Blacks in the United States

This history of medicine and healthcare in the United States is rooted in racism and marked by the mistreatment of Black Americans. These historical structures are woven into modern medicine and their impacts are still felt today. Confronting, naming, and addressing racism, discrimination, and other systemic barriers within the healthcare system must happen to effectively promote health equity.

Racism and Discrimination in Medicine

The history of Black America, including the legacy of slavery and oppression, remains foundational to many health challenges we see today, including segregation, mass incarceration, marginalization, and other influences. The social injustices from racism and discrimination that occurred and that shaped this country, laid the groundwork for poor health outcomes and disparities.

The U.S Public Health Service Syphilis Study at Tuskegee was conducted between 1932 and 1972, to observe and study the natural progression of untreated syphilis on the body.[1] The study ended at the recommendation of an ad hoc advisory panel. Six hundred Black men

---

1 *The US Public Health Study at Tuskegee*, CDC https://www.cdc.gov/tuskegee/index.html

were initially enrolled—300 with latent syphilis and 201 without—and were told they were being treated for "bad blood." The men in this study were misled to believe they were receiving free medical care and researchers disguised placebos as treatment even though penicillin became widely available in 1947. The study lasted for over forty years, was conducted without the benefit of participants' informed consent, and caused the death of 128 of its participants.

In 1951, Henrietta Lacks sought medical care at Johns Hopkins Hospital after complaining of vaginal bleeding.[2] A malignant tumor was found on her cervix, and a sample of her cancer cells was taken without her consent. For years, Lacks's cells, nicknamed HeLa cells, have been cultured and used in experiments to study the effects of toxins, drugs, hormones, and viruses on the growth of cancer cells. Her tissue was patented and has generated millions of dollars in profit for medical researchers, but Lacks's family did not even know the cell cultures existed until more than twenty years after her death.

The history of racism in medicine and the mistreatment of Black Americans was pervasive. Racism was also applicable to Black Americans who aspired to become physicians. The story of Dr. James McCune Smith, who was the first African American physician in the United States is one such powerful example.[3]

Dr. McCune Smith was born into slavery on April 18, 1813, in Manhattan, New York City and was set free on July 4, 1827, at age fourteen, by the Emancipation Act of New York. That was the final date when New York officially freed its remaining slaves. His mother was an enslaved woman named Lavinia who achieved her freedom later in life; in 1855, Smith described her as a "self-emancipated woman."

---

[2] Skloot, Rebecca. *The Immortal Life of Henrietta Lacks*. London: Picador Classic an imprint of Pan MacMillan, 2019.
[3] Morgan, TM. *The Education and Medical Practice* of Dr. James McCune Smith (1813-1865), first black American to hold a medical degree. J Natl Med Assoc. 2003 Jul;95(7):603-14. PMID: 12911258; PMCID: PMC2594637.

As a child, James McCune Smith was a student at the African Free School at No. 2 Mulberry Street. After graduating from the African Free School, Dr. Smith wanted to become a doctor. However, medical schools in the United States did not yet accept students of color. Dr. Smith's applications were denied by numerous American schools. James McCune Smith graduated from the University of Glasgow in Scotland in 1837 and became the first African American to receive a medical degree. During his studies in Glasgow, Smith obtained three university degrees—a bachelor's degree (1835), a master's degree (1836), and his medical doctorate (1837).

After graduating at the top of his class and completing an internship in Paris, Dr. Smith returned to New York in 1837. He opened a pharmacy and medical office that served both Black and White patients, located on 93 West Broadway. As America's first Black doctor, Dr. Smith paved the way for African Americans in the medical field, while committing his life to work for economic and social justice. In addition to his many impressive accomplishments, Dr. Smith also authored the first case report ever written by an African American physician, which discussed opioid use in women. Because of his race, he was not allowed to present the case before the New York Medical and Surgical Society, so Dr. John Watson, who consulted with him on the case, did so instead. The case was eventually published in the *New York Journal of Medicine*. His analytical writing and public lectures had a profound impact on the abolitionist movement and his contributions to medicine opened the door for African Americans in the medical field.

In addition to owning his practice, Dr. Smith was an active abolitionist, educator, and physician. He served as chief physician at the New York City Colored Orphan Asylum and was an accomplished statistician, medical author, and social activist who worked to end slavery. He wrote about medicine, science, education, and racism, and quickly emerged as a powerful anti-slavery lecturer and writer.

Together with abolitionists including Frederick Douglass, Gerrit Smith, and John Brown, he helped found the Radical Abolitionist Party and establish the National Council of the Colored People. His pharmacy also assisted people escaping slavery. Dr. Smith passed away in November of 1865, just a few weeks before slavery was abolished in the United States.

Subsequent books and writings about racism and discrimination in medicine have approached the subject from a historical perspective, and presented the influence of policy or legislative solutions, including the Civil Rights Act of 1964. Among the more noteworthy books are medical ethicist Harriet Washington's critically acclaimed book, *Medical Apartheid: The Dark History of Medical Experimentation on Black Americans from Colonial Times to the Present* (Anchor, 2008). This book traces medical experimentation on Black Americans dating back to the middle of the eighteenth century, culminating with the reporting of the infamous Tuskegee experiment, in which African Americans suffering from syphilis were denied an available cure in order to trace the course of the disease. Washington goes on to investigate medical abuse in research, and finally to address the complex relationship between racism and medicine. Overall, she paints a compelling picture of the history of medical investigations and research on Black Americans.

In her bestselling book, *Just Medicine: A Cure for Racial Inequality in American Healthcare* (NYU Press, 2018), Attorney Dayna Bowen Matthew proposes that the cure for racial and ethnic discrimination in American healthcare lies in reforming the Civil Rights Act of 1964. The question is, can rewriting a failed law lead to better patient outcomes?

An American Health Dilemma: A Medical History of African Americans and the Problem of Race: Beginnings to 1900, by Michael Byrd and Linda Clayton (Routledge, 2000), traces the roots of Western medical bias back to the ancient Egyptian and sub-Saharan practices brought to the New World by slave healers and midwives, then to the Black doctors who broke the color line of nineteenth-century medicine, and finally to the founding of Howard University Medical School in 1867. Then there is the parallel story of the cruelty, neglect, and scientific racism that mark the medical history of the American slave trade and its post-Civil War aftermath.

My Quest for Health Equality: Notes on Learning While Leading (Johns Hopkins Press, 2020), is a memoir by Dr. David Satcher, who has served as director of the Centers for Disease Control and Prevention (CDC), U.S. Surgeon General, and now, director of the National Center for Primary Care. Dr. Satcher is the founder of Satcher Health Leadership Institute at Morehouse College. The book is Satcher's personal story, focusing on his leadership role in resolving national health inequities.

These books are just a handful of the numerous scholarly writings detailing historical racial accounts in medicine and healthcare, and the need for broad policy changes.

Unequal Treatment and COVID-19 Pandemic

The bottom line is that there has been little progress in addressing health disparities for Black Americans since the 2003 Institute of Medicine Report, *Unequal Treatment Confronting Racial and Ethnic Disparities in Healthcare*, which showed that even after adjusting for social determinants of health, such as income, comorbid illness, and various types of health insurance, health outcomes among Blacks were still worse than Whites.

Never have health disparities been so disturbingly apparent as during the COVID-19 epidemic, with the Black population, particularly elderly Black individuals, having the highest death rate.[4] Initially, this death rate disparity was blamed on such reasons as poverty, lack of access to care, lack of health insurance, and various comorbidities,

---
4 Tiffany Ford, Sarah Reber, Richard Reeves Race Gaps in COVID-19 deaths are even bigger than they appear *Brookings Upfront* June 2020 (accessed February 3, 2023)

given the evidence that these are often contributing factors. And yet, the statistics proved otherwise. For the Black population, COVID-19 cut across all socioeconomic statuses.

For example, Prince George's County, a large upper-class Black community in suburban Maryland, led the state in overall cases and ranked second in COVID-19 deaths.[5] Brooklyn, another borough in New York City, which has a 36 percent Black population inclusive of all socioeconomic statuses, had the highest COVID death rates in the city, even though it was home to at least sixteen hospitals and provided readily accessible public transportation to all residents.[6] The sixteen hospitals included three public hospitals where health insurance status was not a requirement to receive healthcare. So, access to care and/or lack of insurance could not be blamed for the high Black mortality rate in either example. Some more disturbing statistics: most employees of the New York City subway system who died from COVID-related deaths were Black with salaries well above the poverty level—approximately $50,000 annually—and had health insurance and pensions. Their deaths were probably the result of being in contact with millions of New Yorkers when COVID was not fully understood. So why did a disproportionate number of Blacks die from COVID? And how can our health systems be modified to prevent such health disparities in the future? The health disparities that were playing out on the ground were not only about economics, lack of access to care, and social determinants of health.

"We still see stark racial disparities even at high income levels," said Dr. Tanjala Purnell, Associate Director of the John Hopkins Center for Health Equity. "People say, 'Oh, minorities are dying

---

[5] Jean Marbella, Naomi Harris Maryland's Prince George's County is among the wealthiest Black communities, but it leads state in coronavirus cases July 2020. *The Baltimore Sun* (accessed February 3, 2023)
[6] Office of the New York State Comptroller Recent trends and impact of COVID-19 in Brooklyn May 2022

because they're poor.' We know that's not the case."[7]

And while there is no evidence that Black Americans are genetically more predisposed to be infected by COVID-19, data from the CDC revealed during the first surge in April 2020 that COVID-19 hospitalization rates among Blacks were 3.3 times the hospitalization rate for Whites[8]. Adding to this alarmingly high death rate for Blacks, it became obvious that the disparities were not only about economics, lack of access to care, social determinants of health, or genetics.

The historic injustices of slavery and oppression, and the structural and systemic racism it has generated and continued to perpetuate, is something that we have long accepted in the US but can no longer afford to continue. They have created the disparities we have today, and disparities are costly. These inequities continue to hold the US back in terms of health rankings among wealthy nations. Ending racial health inequities by addressing the social and economic injustices that sustain them points to the core of our mission. Our history should remind us to keep focus on the health of marginalized groups, with an appreciation toward improving the health of all. In today's America, health disparities and inequities in health outcomes are in full view.

There is another dimension to America's health disparities beyond contribution from the social determinants of health. It has to do with human value. The lack of human value is currently pervasive in health institutions, particularly as it relates to African Americans, and that lack of human value has direct, negative impacts on their

---

[7] Jean Marbella, Naomi Harris Maryland's Prince George's County is among the wealthiest Black communities, but it leads the state in coronavirus case as of July 2020. *The Baltimore Sun* (accessed February 3, 2023)

[8] Romano SD, Blackstock AJ, Taylor EV, et al. *Trends in Racial and Ethnic Disparities in COVID-19 Hospitalizations, by Region—United States, March—December 2020*. MMWR Morb Mortal Wkly Rep 2021;70:560—565. Romano, Sebastian D., Anna J. Blackstock, Ethel V. Taylor, Suad El Burai Felix, Stacey Adjei, Christa-Marie Singleton, Jennifer Fuld, Beau B. Bruce, and Tegan K. Boehmer. "Trends in Racial and Ethnic Disparities in Covid-19 Hospitalizations, by Region — United States, March—December 2020." *MMWR. Morbidity and Mortality Weekly Report* 70, no. 15 (April 16, 2021): 560—65. https://doi.org/10.15585/mmwr.mm7015e2.

health outcomes. The incomprehensible, inhumane killing of George Floyd, the impact of COVID-19, and persisting poor health outcomes, particularly for the Black community, caused me to reflect on my internship and residency training in Internal Medicine at Harlem Hospital/Columbia Presbyterian. Under the leadership of Dr. Gerald Thomson, then Director of Medicine, the expectation was that all patients were valuable human beings, and all were expected to receive the best healthcare irrespective of their socioeconomic status, race, gender, religious affiliation, or other characteristics that are often stigmatized, such as opioid addiction.

The intent of the nine simple solutions that will be outlined in my book, will add an additional dimension to achieving health equity with a focus on the patient voices and the common thread: the human experience—the absence of patient engagement, and how prioritizing and centering these issues can lead to better health outcomes.

CHAPTER 2

Harlem on My Mind

As I look back, we were Afro-wearing Black and long-haired anti-Vietnam war-protesting White doctors-in-training with the shared understanding and expectation to get our patients well by the morning report that occurred the next day. There were no racial tensions or conflicts. In the cafeteria, Black and White doctors were seated together and the only pattern of segregation, if any, was due to shared identities of the entry medical training class, such as being interns, residents, or chief residents.

We came from all over the country; north, south, east, and west, urban, suburban, and rural areas of the country and from Ivy League and non-Ivy League medical schools. Collectively, we came to Harlem Hospital not because we had to, but because we chose to. We were eager to experience the new Harlem Renaissance.

The collective brain power there was off the charts. One moment comes to mind when I look back on my time with my colleagues. A few of us interns were at lunch, and we all noticed that Keith had a letter in his hand and a look of pride on his face. "What's going on?" we asked, as he sat there with his eyes buried in the letter and his smile growing with every moment.

He was from Arkansas. His family, along with the entire Black community there, were farmers. When he was accepted to Harvard

Medical School, everyone in his community was so proud of him that they got together and collected one hundred dollars in his honor. Now, here he was, pursuing his residency at Harlem Hospital, sitting at the table with this letter in his hands, and with the look of pride growing by the moment.

And there we all were, trying to figure out what was in the letter.

Finally, he said to us, "My father was made the first Black postman."

"You mean he was made head of the post office?" one of us asked, because most individuals that were delivering mail in New York were Black, and becoming a postman was no big deal. Not in New York.

No, he told us. It turned out that his father was the first Black man in his hometown in Arkansas to get a job as a mailman delivering the mail. He was so proud of his father. I will never forget that moment. That's when I got to appreciate the similarities and variations in societal struggles for African Americans based on geographic location.

Medical Training at Harlem Hospital

Harlem Hospital Center, branded as NYC H+H/Harlem, is a 272-bed, public teaching hospital affiliated with Columbia University. It is located at 506 Lenox Avenue in Harlem, Manhattan, New York City.[9]

When Harlem Hospital Center opened its doors on April 18, 1887, it was located at the juncture of East 120th Street and the East River. The Hospital was a former Victorian mansion lit with ornate gas fixtures and heated by marble fireplaces. The Hospital's initial purpose was to serve as a reception center for patients awaiting transfer to Ward's and Randall's Islands. It also served as an emergency branch of Bellevue Hospital, providing both ambulance and hospital service.

The hospital assumed part of its present site on the east side of Lenox Avenue between 136th and 137th Streets in 1907, where it opened as a

---

[9] Harlem Hospital Center https://www.nychealthandhospitals.org/locations/harlem/ Accessed July 2023 "NYC Health + Hospitals/Harlem." NYC Health + Hospitals, August 23, 2023. https://www.nychealthandhospitals.org/locations/harlem/.

150-bed facility. From 1907 to 1960 several expansion programs were completed, including a 390-bed expansion and a Nurses Residence in 1915; in 1935, the Women's Pavilion was constructed, adding 282 additional beds, and the Nurses Residence was expanded. In 1944, the Pediatrics Building was constructed, and in 1950, the Samuel Kountz Pavilion, a 233-bed acute and outpatient facility was constructed. The original 150-bed hospital was replaced in the late 1960s by the eighteen-story Martin Luther King, Jr. Pavilion. In 1998, the Ronald H. Brown Ambulatory Care Pavilion was completed. Harlem Hospital Center has a long and respected reputation as an educator of Black health professionals. Although Black physicians were not appointed to the medical staff in any significant number until 1927, minority physicians have since come to dominate the medical faculty and residency training programs. Today, the hospital is a primary resource for medical practice and education for a heterogeneous mixture of professionals who are pursuing careers in healthcare and are dedicated to service in medically underserved areas.[10]

The hospital is a member of the NYC H+H/Harlem, formerly known as New York City Health and Hospitals Corporation and the Generations+/Northern Manhattan Health Network.[11]

Achievements

Harlem Hospital has received numerous awards. In 2000, the hospital received the Healthcare Association of New York State Community Health Improvement Award, given in honor of the hospital's Injury Prevention Program. The injury center at the hospital was recognized

---

10 Harlem Hospital Center. Our History https://www.cumc.columbia.edu/harlem-hospital/about/history accessed July 2023 "Our History." Vagelos College of Physicians and Surgeons, November 8, 2023. https://www.vagelos.columbia.edu/education/residencies-fellowships-and-training/harlem-hospital-center/about-harlem-hospital-center/our-history.
11 Harlem Hospital https://www.nychealthandhospitals.org/locations/harlem/ Accessed July 2023 "NYC Health + Hospitals/Harlem." NYC Health + Hospitals, August 23, 2023. https://www.nychealthandhospitals.org/locations/harlem/.

for targeting window falls, violent injuries, and bicycle injuries.

In 1958, Harlem Hospital was credited with saving the life of Dr. Martin Luther King, Jr. after a woman described to be emotionally and mentally disturbed stabbed him in the chest at Blumstein's Department Store on 125th Street, where he had just finished giving a speech at a book signing. Harlem's Chief of Surgery Dr. Aubrey Maynard used the thoracic surgical procedure that he developed along with his team, consisting of Dr. John Cordice and Dr. Emil Naclerio, performed the innovative surgery to remove the knife blade, which was millimeters from Dr. King's aorta. In 1963, in part because of the successful surgery, Dr. King was able to give his "I have a Dream Speech" in Washington. This remains a point of pride for Harlem Hospital and the greater Harlem community.

My beginnings in the ICU

I will never forget my first day at Harlem Hospital. The date was July 1, 1978, and there were thirty of us feeling both excited and overwhelmed as we embarked on our first day of internship in Internal Medicine. I parked in the lot across the street from the hospital, walked to the entrance of the emergency department (ED), then exited to the main lobby, where I took the elevator to the Intensive Care Unit (ICU) on the 15th floor for my first rotation. After a brief meeting with the chief resident to hear what was expected of us, I found myself on call for the first time. It was my responsibility to assess each patient admitted to the ICU and determine their medical status and provide excellent medical care. If it hadn't been for Nurse Betty, I don't know what I would have done that day.

The ICU was an intimidating place to start on the first day of my internship. There were three divisions of the intensive care units: general ICU, respiratory ICU, and the coronary care unit (CCU). I was in the respiratory unit when my first page came through from CCU, which was right next door. The patient was a sixty-year-old woman complaining of chest pains. I will never forget the look on Nurse Betty's face when I entered the room. She was the nurse in charge of the CCU. She had a quiet presence, but one can be quiet and still scare the daylights out of people. And there I was, the first of the new interns she would be dealing with that day. And she did her sarcastic best to help me with my first patient, as I was terrified of making a mistake.

"Do you want to examine the patient?" she said. "I think you do."

"Do you want to start an IV? I thought so."

"Do you want to look at the EKG? I thought so."

She was telling me what I was supposed to be doing step by step. At this point, knowing that the patient was not having a heart attack but was experiencing a heart arrhythmia, Nurse Betty again looked at me and said, "Do you want to give her some lidocaine? I think you do." She then handed me the syringe that she had already prepared.

It was not until after my patient was stabilized and doing well that Nurse Betty said, "Oh my God, here we go again. It's July," as she knew she would be overseeing new, inexperienced interns for months to come.

And at the end of each month, we all wound up hugging her. "Oh, get away from me," she would say to each of us, but in a kind way.

She cared about us, and she cared about the patients. So began my clinical indoctrination as a physician to provide excellent care at Harlem Hospital.

Dr. Gerald E. Thomson, who had grown up in Harlem, was the first Black Director of Medicine at Harlem Hospital. Prior to his arrival in 1971, 99 percent of the patients were Black, and 90 percent of the residents were White, and came from Bellevue Hospital, and the disease mortality rate of patients was among the highest in the country. That was all destined to change, but Rome wasn't built in a day.

New York City Commissioner of Health and former Harlem Hospital resident Mary Bassett recalled in an interview with *Columbia*

Medicine what Dr. Thomson was up against when he arrived and how he built what needed to happen:

> We lacked supplies, we had very sick patients, the operating room would be shut down because they didn't have air conditioning, and I remember the night they ran out of respirators. But despite those daunting conditions, Dr. Thomson inspired us all by his example, generating standards, demanding quality of care, and commanding respect. For a whole generation of physicians who trained at Harlem Hospital, he exemplified what it meant to be a physician dedicated to community.[12]

Dr. Thomson's expectation of excellence influenced every new intern and resident, as recollected by Dr. David Savage when he spoke at the 2017 Harlem Hospital reunion honoring Dr. Thomson. "He was there because this hospital was standing in central Harlem, and he believed profoundly that all human beings, be they poor or disadvantaged, deserved compassionate and high-quality medical care as much as anybody else."

Indeed, Rome wasn't built in a day. But it was being rebuilt. Dr. Thomson's attitude was that we were going to get these patients well. He had no bias as to who the patient was, whether the individual was working or unemployed, went to church or not, or was addicted to drugs or not.

Get the Patient Well by Morning Report

The statement, "Get the patient well by morning report," was embedded in our brains by the chief residents.

---

[12] Gerald Thomson: The Breadth of a Physician's Commitments. Columbia Medicine Alumni Profile. By Peter Wortsman. http://columbiamedicinemagazine.org/alumni-news-notes/fall-2018/alumni-profile Wortsman, Peter. "Alumni Profile." Columbia Medicine Magazine, May 29, 2019. https://columbiamedicinemagazine.org/alumni-news-notes/fall-2018/alumni-profile.

Morning report was a standard morning event. As an intern, if you were on call the day before, all admitted patients on a unit, be it one or five, had to be presented to the attending physician responsible for the medical unit where an intern was located. First, we had to present the reason *or reasons* why the patient came to the emergency room: the symptoms, vital signs, physical exam, any labs or X-rays done in the ED, diagnosis, and reason for admission. The patient's social history had to be comprehensive. It needed to include detailed information on who the individual was, in terms of marital status, living arrangements, employment status, religion, any substance use or addiction issues including smoking, alcohol, or drugs. Once the patient was admitted to the unit, the plan of care, treatment delivered, results, and the patient's improvement were discussed at Morning Report. Even though there was a significant problem with drug overdose and substance use addiction, a comprehensive social history was the norm. It was unacceptable for a social history to be limited to non-smoker or non-drinker without including information about their living arrangement or educational background for example. Sadly, a comprehensive social history tends to be absent in most patients' social history in today's medical records.

Regardless of how ill each patient presented, it was a mandate to maximize the possibility of improving their health status. We were expected to provide excellent care irrespective of obstacles, and as a result, improve the health of the Harlem community. And that was embedded in our brains from day one.

A major added value was understanding the role of religion in the population and the complexity of a historical perspective. One patient in particular, has always stood out in my mind as manifesting the importance of the role of religion.

Role of Religion: Sunday in Harlem

It was Sunday morning and I had just entered her room. Recently admitted, in her sixties, she was sitting calmly in her bed with her Bible in hand. Upon seeing me, she closed the Bible and put it in her lap. I told her that I was her doctor.

"No, you are not," she shot back.

Perhaps she was confused and thought another physician would be taking care of her, so I reassured her that I was her doctor.

"No, you are not," she stated even more vehemently. "God is taking care of me today, and so now you have time to go to church and praise God."

I remember thinking, "How do I compete with God?"

As an intern on call, you cannot leave the hospital to go anywhere, including church. Like an idiot, I repeated myself. She just looked at me, opened her Bible, looked at me again and then looked at the door. As if to say, "Don't let the door hit you on the way out."

Lesson learned: The importance of combining clinical care with the recognition of the importance of religion in the Black population—priceless.

Another case that I will never forget occurred on another Sunday in Harlem. The patient was a female in her sixties who had been admitted to the Coronary Care Unit (CCU) for chest pains. An hour earlier, she had been in church and complained of chest pain and dizziness, and now she was here with all her church friends wanting to come into the CCU to see and pray with her. And I was the one who had to go tell them, "No, you can't all come in. Just one family member," to which they replied, "We're all God's family."

So, I went to the patient in her room and told her that a lot of people from the church were in the hallway at the entrance of the CCU wanting to see her. "If you'll just tell me the name of your immediate family, I can have that person come in to visit with you," to which she reiterated, "We're all God's family."

Key cultural patient stories

As an intern and as a resident at Harlem Hospital, I did not just learn how to provide excellent clinical care, I learned about various concerns that patients had because of our African American history. Such was the case with one patient who was perhaps my single most important learning experience at Harlem, where the severity of the patient's illness and his cultural history crossed. I was not prepared for that. It had to do with the cultural challenges of being an African American and the need to understand our history, for without this history and the ability to put it into perspective it will unfairly define who we are as patients and as a people.

I was a first-year resident on call when the emergency room contacted me about an admission. I went down to the ER and transported the patient to his room. He had been admitted for diabetic ketoacidosis (DKA), which occurs when the body does not produce enough insulin to metabolize sugar and so it must turn to breaking down fat for energy. The result is a buildup of acids in the bloodstream called ketones, leading to diabetic ketoacidosis, which can lead to death.

In those days, interns and residents transported patients from the emergency room upstairs to the unit to which they were assigned. The assigned nurse then helped me to place him in his bed. I then left and went to the nursing station to read his admission information and to determine his severity of illness comparison when he presented to the Emergency Department (ED), treatment given, and his current health status while the nurse was performing her nursing duties, including taking his vital signs.

Shortly thereafter, I returned to the patient's room to continue the treatment protocol for DKA and found his bed empty. I checked with the nurse who was assigned to him. She was as surprised as I was that he wasn't in his bed. I was concerned that he had perhaps gone to the bathroom and passed out, since he had a severe illness.

We both went to the men's bathroom, but he was not there.

That is when my panic set in. I ran to the elevator to see if he had left against medical advice. Running toward the elevator, I had to pass the patient lounge. I stopped, looked in, and there he was, sitting watching television with a bunch of other patients and nurses taking the patients' blood pressure.

I begged him to come back to his room. He didn't even look at me. His eyes were glued to the television. I explained to him that he had a very severe medical problem that could be life-threatening. I was literally trembling, with my voice going up a notch, and I told him that he was putting his life in danger. Still no response. I called the nurse to take his vital signs and check his blood sugar, all while he just sat there, glued to the TV, adamant and angry. He finally stated in no uncertain terms, "I didn't want to come to the hospital in the first place," he fumed, "but my wife made me. I've been waiting all this time to find out where I came from and who I am, and I'm not leaving."

He stuck his hand out while sitting and glued to the television. He was vehement while not looking at me and stated, "Treat me here, I am not leaving."

I had no clue what he was talking about, why the lounge was packed, or why they were all glued to the TV while nurses took their blood pressure. That's when I looked at the television and suddenly understood. Everyone was watching the TV mini-series *Roots*. It was a defining moment. Kunta Kinte was an African who came to the United States involuntarily due to the slave trade. He was being whipped multiple times because he would not say that his name was Toby. It was part of his indoctrination into his new slave culture, and he would have nothing to do with it. He just kept repeating when asked the question while being whipped repeatedly, "What's your name?" He responded "Kunta Kinte."

When he was finally whipped into submission, he said his name was Toby, and the emotions and sadness that filled the room was palpable. The tears were tearing at all our hearts. I remember my patient in tears walking directly in front of the TV and saying, "Your name is not Toby; it will always be Kunta Kinte. Don't you ever forget it."

I gave him a tissue, and at that point he was willing to go back to his room. With continuous treatment, his DKA was resolved before the morning report. It was clear to me that he had manifested not only the pain and suffering that we as a people endured against all odds, but also the absence of African American cultural history, which is not taught in medical schools, as well as the lack of mental health counseling for African American atrocity survivors.

That was the key and is often still the missing element today. Dr. Thomson summed it up in 2017 at the reunion at Harlem Hospital honoring him when again we all came from north, south, east, and west in recognition of what he had taught us with one phrase: "Understanding the value of human rights in delivering healthcare, and who we are as physicians and human beings."

For me, the training at Harlem Hospital was the road to understanding the crossroads between the delivery of excellent healthcare and the roles that history, culture, and religion play in the Black community. After all these professional lessons, my learning experience was about to take a more personal turn.

CHAPTER 3

Queens Health Network: Care Management Program Ahead of its Time

In 2007, after two decades as a primary care physician in community health centers where I grew up in the Bronx, memories of my medical training at Harlem Hospital were embedded in my brain as I accepted the position as Associate Executive Director of Care Management at New York City Health and Hospitals (NYC H+H) Queens Health Network (QHN), which includes Elmhurst and Queens Hospitals. It was as if I was back home at NYC Health + Hospital even though it was not at Harlem Hospital.

NYC Health + Hospitals is the nation's largest municipal healthcare delivery system in the United States includes eleven acute care hospitals, ambulatory care facilities, long-term care facilities, community health centers, school health programs, rehab facilities, and a health plan MetroPlus. The health system provides essential services to more than 1.4 million New Yorkers every year in more than seventy patient care locations and in their homes. In-patient hospital visits are over a million, ambulatory care visits 900,000 and 18,000 births. Central Office is inclusive of and not limited to the C-Suite administration, legal, quality, patient experience officer, medical and professional affairs, human resources, and finance.

I was hired in 2007 by Dr. Ann Sullivan, Senior Vice President (SVP) of Queens Health Network located in the borough of Queens, New York City. Dr. Sullivan was ahead of her time in terms of recognizing the need to develop a Care Management program for both hospitals. After several interviews with CEOs of both Elmhurst and Queens hospital, Chief Medical Officers and then jointly and individually with medical and administrative directors of services including the emergency department, inpatient, and ambulatory care. I was hired shortly thereafter and assumed the role of Associate Executive Director of Care Management. One of my responsibilities was to develop and implement what would be the first Care Management program in NYC Health + Hospitals on the adult medical services.

QHN has a unique healthcare system serving the largest and most ethnically diverse communities in New York City and has affiliations with Mount Sinai School of Medicine, New York University, and Columbia Presbyterian Hospital. Elmhurst Hospital is a Level One trauma center with 545 beds, and Queens Hospital has 261 beds, both with multiple specialties including behavioral health and ambulatory care centers.

The Queens Hospital patient population was predominantly Black with a significant Guyanese Indian population, and Elmhurst was more diverse and included a large Hispanic, Indian, Chinese, and a growing Russian population. The Black population at Elmhurst was relatively small when compared to Queens Hospital.

Bridge Team Concept

In 2007, Care Management was a new concept that not many in the medical profession were aware of. I requested and collected Queens and Elmhurst Hospital data, including race and ethnicity data, ED visits, in-patient admissions, and top diagnosis related to readmission. I had conversations with directors of service divisions along with medical, nursing, and social work staff as well as hospital CEOs and board members about Care Management processes. Based on the data collected and a considerable number of interviews, I wrote a Care Management Concept paper that demonstrated sustainable processes whose essence was based on collaboration between patients and families, the clinical teams in the ED, inpatient, and transition to ambulatory care and communities. I ensured that we recognized and appreciated the cultural diversity of the communities served. The program was approved in all its aspects by the Chief Financial Officer and the Care Management process was implemented at both Elmhurst and Queens Hospitals.

A key individual who was involved in the rollout of the Care Management processes at both Elmhurst and Queens Hospitals was Prajakta Vagal, Director of Care Management, who reported to me directly and was responsible for data collection, analysis, and implementation monitoring. I think without Prajakta, the rollout and sustainability of the processes would have been limited.

At the heart of the Care Management program at both hospitals was a unique feature "The Bridge Team," whose responsibility was to bridge the gaps in care from the ED, inpatient, and transition to ambulatory care and community for complicated high-risk patients and families inclusive of individuals with Sickle Cell Disease (SCD) by addressing their life-threatening health challenges without being judgmental.

The idea of the Bridge Team was to facilitate the collaboration between the clinical teams, patients, caregivers, and their families, resolve their concerns, communicate information promptly, and support the transition of patients to the appropriate level of care.

The Bridge Team consisted of directors of Care Management of both hospitals, who reported to me, and nurse care managers in the emergency department, inpatient, and ambulatory care, who reported to the director of Care Management and social workers.

At Queen's Hospital, one of the most vulnerable patient populations in my opinion, were individuals with Sickle Cell Disease (SCD), a genetic disorder that affects red blood cells. The disease is characterized by the production of abnormal hemoglobin (termed sickled red blood cells), resulting in anemia, susceptibility to infections such as pneumococcal pneumonia, stroke, and multiple organ dysfunction. SCD is a life-threatening, inherited blood disorder affecting more than 100,000 Americans. This is an approximate number reported by the CDC, since the exact number is unknown. Painful vaso-occlusive crises, the hallmark of this disease, result in substantial suffering from chronic pain, leading to associated stigma as drug-seeking. Without adequate treatment, the disease affects all organs and is associated with decreased quality of life and a shortened life span. All babies in the US regardless of ethnicity are tested for SCD as part of newborn screening. It is thus important to recognize this disease is a common and important medical condition among Americans with ancestry in tropical regions where malaria is endemic. Thus, the disease does not affect just Black Americans. Individuals of Mediterranean, Middle Eastern, Indian, and Latino descent are also affected. The causative mutation in SCD primarily arose on the African continent because of the protective effect of the carrier state against malaria, so most patients have a shared African ancestry. As a result, it is assumed that the disease largely affects those of African ancestry.

Although it's a disorder affecting people of all races globally, in the United States, as a direct result of the transatlantic slave trade, nearly all patients are Black. It affects one out of every 365 African Americans born in America and about 1 in 12 carry the Sickle Cell trait.[13] SCD also occurs in about one out of every 16,300 Hispanic

---

13 Newborn screening for Sickle Cell Diseases in the United States: A review of data spanning 2 decades. Therrell BL Jr, Lloyd-Puryear MA, Eckman JR, Mann MY. Semin Perinatol. 2015 Apr;39(3):238-51. Therrell, Bradford L., Michele A. Lloyd-Puryear, James R. Eckman, and Marie Y. Mann. "Newborn Screening for Sickle Cell Diseases in the United States: A Review of Data Spanning 2 Decades." *Seminars in Perinatology* 39, no. 3 (April 2015): 238—51. https://doi.org/10.1053/j.semperi.2015.03.008.

births. This fact would be mere medical trivia if we did not live in such a highly racialized society.

Individuals diagnosed with SCD often receive a lower standard of care, and race does play a role in these disparities across health systems, regardless of geographic location. Families with children with SCD love their pediatrician and adolescent physicians but when they get to adult care, they are the most vilified and least engaged patients. Once they become adults, they are potentially midway through their life expectancy.

Stop-in-your-tracks moment.

The unexpected is what I refer to as a "Stop-in-your-tracks moment." Those moments were extremely enlightening, inspirational, and humbling and caused me to continuously reassess my knowledge base and the implementation of multiple unique system processes that I designed while serving as Associate Executive Director of Care/Case management.

The Care Management Program with nursing care managers in the emergency room and inpatient and ambulatory care service provided added nursing staff that enhanced collaboration with the ED directors of both hospitals that were pivotal in achieving positive outcomes at both hospitals.

The job of the Bridge Team, as stated earlier was to bridge the gap in care for whatever reason and as a result, an eighteen-year-old patient with SCD was referred to the Bridge Team. She had a reputation for having an attitude, was disrespectful, and had a significant amount of ED visits and readmissions.

As the Bridge Team and I were about to enter her room, I saw a young woman, still in her teens, talking on her phone. She glanced up at me and held my gaze, her eyes angry and defiant. "I'm on the phone," she snapped, as if I, the doctor, were an intruder in her bedroom.

The team began whispering, stating that her behavior was so attitudinal and disrespectful. I remember my statement to the team;

namely, "Which eighteen-year-old does not have an attitudinal behavior even without a life-threatening disease? Let's give her the benefit of the doubt and wait until she is off her phone."

When she put her phone down and we were about to enter her room, she stated in no uncertain terms, "If you have a cure for my disease, come in and talk to me, if you don't keep walking."

Suddenly, I was the child, and she was the adult as she stated with piercing eyes, "Did you hear what I said? I am going to repeat it one more time," and she did. It sounded like a statement that I would say to my children when they were not following directions.

I was caught off guard by her very deliberate and intentional statement. For a moment, I did not know how to respond, and as I gathered my thoughts, I responded and said, "No, I don't have a cure, but let me think about what you said, and I will come back and speak with you later."

Clearly, a major stop-in-my-tracks moment!

Later that evening, I returned to her room with the intent of getting to know her as an individual as opposed to who she was perceived to be. I entered her room, and she was receptive and did not project the image that I was an intruder. She was calm and receptive, and introduced me to who she really was. It was then I learned that two years prior, at age sixteen, her mother was going to work when she developed chest pains on the bus and was taken to an emergency room, where she died of a heart attack. The previous year, at age seventeen, her sister had been admitted to a hospital for Sickle Cell crisis and sepsis and died in the intensive care unit. At that point, we both teared up and hugged each other.

This individual was amazing, intellectual, and analytical, particularly for her age. Who they perceived her to be was not the reality of who she really was. She made another powerful statement and calmly educated me when she stated, "You doctors don't teach me about Sickle Cell, Sickle Cell teaches me." There was a moment of silence as I had to gather my breath and my emotions as a mom, physician, and an African American human being. I followed up by asking if she had been given a depression screening or been referred to a psychologist, and she replied, "No."

It was the emotional meeting with her and hearing her voice that evening that was the motivation in my decision to start the first Sickle Cell Support Group at New York City Health & Hospitals/Queens. It was all about creating an environment where patients could voice who they were, their fears, concerns about the care and treatment they received, as well as personal and family issues, their recommendations, and whatever else they wanted to share with the group about having this horrific, unimaginably painful disease.

Sickle Cell Support Group

In collaboration with the Emergency Department Director, I implemented the ED protocol that assigned that physicians or physician assistants should provide needed care in an empathetic and non-judgmental manner for patients with Sickle Cell disease, including the elimination of the term "drug seeker," which was not supported by medical literature. Most individuals with Sickle Cell disease in the US are African American/Black population. They have two types of severe pain: The unimaginable physical pain associated with their Sickle Cell crisis and the mental and emotional pain when one is referred to as a "drug seeker." The mental and emotional pain is avoidable, but the physical pain is not, as it is a complication of the disease. The mental and emotional pain that an individual suffers while accessing care to eliminate the severity of physical pain during a crisis episode is unwarranted, unnecessary, lacks compassion and empathy, and is a result of either conscious or unconscious bias toward this population.

The ED nurse care manager was assigned to contact hematology and primary care physicians to notify them that their patient was in the ED and would be admitted or discharged, and/or need a follow-up appointment.

The care manager's role was also to discuss with patients about joining The Sickle Cell Support Group and its purpose. If they agreed, the care manager would provide a list of potential attendees to the director of Care Management and follow up with the assigned date and time for the support group meeting.

The support group would meet at noon once per week before the hematology clinic. Lunch was provided. The participating staff included a psychologist, social worker, inpatient care manager, director of Care Management, and me. Usually, the number of patients ranged from ten to fifteen individuals. The support group meetings were unscripted because we wanted the individuals to determine what they wanted to discuss, their concerns, their fears, aspirations, and recommendations. We implemented a survey for the support group participants because I thought it was important to understand how the individual participants felt about their medical condition, their experiences in the ED, and perspectives about their hospitalization. We also felt it was important to solicit information about issues they felt might need to be addressed to help improve their care and health outcomes.

Patient Stories from Queen's Sickle Cell Support Group

In our first meeting, I was blown away by the emotional truth that was shared during the support group listening sessions. Below are some of the statements that were made by the patients.

Patient Voices included phrases such as: "I hate my mom!" As a mom, I was traumatized by the statement. I asked, "Why do you hate your mom?" She responded in a communicative way and with a certain degree of comfort with her response, "I don't hate her now, that was when I was younger. Back then I never understood why she sided with the doctors in keeping me in pain; why didn't they just let me die. As I got older, I knew she loved me beyond the moon and wanted more than anything for me to live pain-free."

Another patient's powerful responses when we were discussing the trauma of being referred to as a drug seeker. "Yes, I am a drug seeker. I need drugs to relieve my pain. But I am not just seeking drugs.

One patient noted: "The pain is like a sledgehammer constantly hitting me up and down my spine. When I'm in crisis, the pain is so severe that I really want to die. When I am home and feeling better, these thoughts go away."

Others made statements such as: "I often ask myself, 'Why me God?' and realize there are no answers."; "I have goals and aspirations despite this disease." Another disheartening comment was from a patient who said "I have a 50 percent chance when admitted to a hospital that someone will be nice to me. Why did it take so long to recognize us? Is it because of who we are?"

These were powerful, eye-opening statements.

This next story sheds an insightful view and perspective on the interactions between siblings when one has the disease, and the other does not. The sibling without SCD was her brother and was on the school's basketball team. The team's history of competition was that they were always eliminated during the first round. However, that year her brother's team made it to the semifinals, and the next day they would be playing to be in the finals. Needless to say, her brother was over the moon with excitement as was she, her mom, and dad, as this was a moment that had never happened before. Sadly, at around 1 a.m. that morning, a Sickle Cell crisis reared its ugly head and their dad drove his wife and his daughter to the hospital, and her brother had to go to the once-in-a-lifetime moment in his basketball career at the time by himself. I can just imagine the sense of guilt she felt, probably more than once, when her disease superseded her brother's presence and accomplishments.

I hope that this story will shed a light on the need for family counseling for individuals with SCD, and for anyone that this story resonates with.

Myths and Facts from Support Group

The support groups gave patients with Sickle Cell disease and their caregivers an opportunity to share their experiences and recommend needed changes that health systems could do to improve their lives and health outcomes.

As part of the support group activities, I developed and administered a survey to participants to obtain their perspective of issues that they thought might help improve their care and health outcomes.

Sickle support group survey

Survey for a Sickle Cell Support Group—to be administered to the group.

General questions:

What is your country of birth? What is your parent's country of birth?
Are you employed? If employed, did you finish high school/college/other?
Do you have children with Sickle Cell disease?
Language (primary) spoken.

English_____Spanish_____French_____Other (please specify)_____
Recommendations to hospital staff and physician (optional)_____

How often during the year, do you have pain requiring an emergency room visit?

- Do you think that the care you receive in the emergency room addresses your needs?
- How effective does the staff control your pain in the ED?
- How many times per year do you get hospitalized?
- During your ED visit or hospitalization do you feel the doctors listen to you?
- Have you ever been called a drug seeker?

- How did it make you feel?
- Do you have a primary care physician?
- Are you followed in the pain management clinic and hematology clinic?
- Do you feel depressed?
- Do you receive ongoing mental health counseling?

The Sickle Cell Patient Support Group helped to change the negative perceptions to embrace the reality about who these individual human beings are. They taught us about who they were and encouraged us to understand their fears and learn what was important to them and to acknowledge that they had dreams and aspirations like any other human being, as well. The words "drug seekers" were never used going forward.

The Bridge Teams of both hospitals were major contributors to decreasing inpatient readmissions, ED visits, and more sustainable transition care. To this day, treatment of patients with Sickle Cell disease are a priority at Queens Hospital. I recently spoke with the Queens Hospital Emergency Department Director who was very instrumental in the success of the Care Management initiative concerning Sickle Cell patients. He stated that readmission was significantly down, patient engagement and collaboration were up, and contentiousness between staff and patients has been eliminated. Currently, there is a physician's assistant assigned for all emergency visits, and the use of the observation unit has proven to be effective.

I reached out to various Sickle Cell organizations across several states to inquire about resources in place, and no one I spoke with admitted to having an adult sickle support group. In addition, I inquired whether depression screening was done at various doctor's visits, and whether referral to a mental health counselor for individuals and or family counseling services was offered where needed. The majority of the doctors I spoke with, said "No."

Individuals diagnosed with SCD receive a lower standard of care, and racism does play a role in these disparities. Unfortunately, the social construct of race in America requires the majority of patients with SCD not only to face the consequences of a life-threatening health condition, but also to navigate a society in which the color of their skin is often an unfair disadvantage, and which causes them to be labeled as "drug seekers."

Medical evidence does not support the use of the term "drug seeker" when a patient with Sickle Cell crisis is requesting a higher dose of an opioid medication, and that the medication be administered intravenously. Such a patient knows from experience what they need to get them through the unimaginable pain crisis, and they are often under-medicated when those treating them misperceive them as "drug seekers," which is, sadly, the perception across a large majority of health systems nationally. When a patient is misperceived as being a "drug seeker," poor health outcomes can become the accepted norm.

The notion that patients with SCD are "drug seekers" and that they are the most addicted of any patient population is the national perception among healthcare providers and health systems. These patients are, in fact, the least addicted of any group with chronic pain syndrome. This has been documented in the medical literature. They are the least addicted but the most vilified.

Myth	Fact
Sickle Cell patients have a higher degree of drug addiction than the general population.	Opioid addiction for Sickle Cell patients ranges from 0.5 to 8 percent vs. 3 to 16 percent in patients with other chronic pain syndromes. Reference: Zempsky, William T. "Treatment of Sickle Cell Pain." JAMA 302, no. 22 (2009): 2479. https://doi.org/10.1001/jama.2009.1811.

Behaviors often described in patients with SCD, such as requesting a specific dose of opioid or requesting that the opioid be administered intravenously, may be normative in patients who have experienced a history of under-treatment of pain; less indicative of abuse than behaviors such as illicit drug use or using opioids for symptoms other than pain.

Lessons learned from Sickle Cell Support Group sessions and discussion

1. Improving patient trust is crucial to improving the lives of individuals with this horrible life-threatening disease.
2. Trust starts with a patient engagement philosophy that is nonjudgmental.
3. An effective transition of care process is important to patients and their families.
4. Partnering with community-based organizations is crucial to helping the patients in the broader context of the individual.
5. SCD, like other chronic diseases, does not have to control one's life.
6. Patients should make every attempt to control the disease and not have the disease control them.

In the words of Dr. William T. Zempsky, a leading pain researcher, "Difficult patients are not just born, they are in part created by their passage through the medical system. Not only has this system failed to cure them, but it may also have done unpleasant things to make matters worse."

For all hospitals that treat individuals with SCD, I strongly recommend implementation of the following processes for adult patients:

Key Implementation Processes for Adult Patients with Sickle Cell Disease

1. Establishment of a Sickle Cell Patient Support Group inclusive of patients in the ED, ambulatory care, and those admitted to the hospital.
2. Providing healthcare in a nonjudgmental manner coupled with organizational cultural competence. The organizational cultural competence needs to be inclusive and include efforts to dismantle negative perception or stereotypes about who the individual really is.
3. Ensuring personalized Transition Care plans from adolescent to adult care

Patients with Sickle Cell Disease: Conversations with Physicians and the Clinical Care Team

Examples of questions and comments for patients and their families if they are in the emergency department, and they are not getting the needed care they deserve.

- I am a human being who happens to be African American.
- I have a life-threatening disorder, Sickle Cell disease.
- I am in severe pain, and I need to be valued and treated Now!
- Like you, I have dreams and aspirations, so please do not cut my life short because you don't value me.
- If no response, ask to speak with the ED Director.
- If you are experiencing a painful crisis, and you are unable to speak, have a family member speak for you.
- If you don't have a PCP or a Hematologist, upon discharge from the ED, make sure you have a referral to a hematologist and PCP.

If you are hospitalized, ask to speak to a behavioral health specialist.

- A behavioral health specialist is helpful for discussing your feelings, fears, anxiety, depression, family circumstances, and anything that's important to you.
- Make sure you have a follow-up appointment on discharge.
- You don't have to feel uncomfortable requesting a mental health counselor.
- It should be a vital part of your treatment for SCD.
- Recognized as a need in other life-threatening diseases such as Cystic Fibrosis; so why not SCD?

Important Statement
Keep this statement below in your phone.

In the words of Dr. William T. Zempsky, a leading pain researcher, "Difficult patients are not just born; they are in part created by their passage through the medical system. Not only has this system failed to cure them, but it may also have done unpleasant things to make matters worse."

1. Zempsky, William T. "Treatment of Sickle Cell Pain." JAMA 302, no. 22 (2009):2479. https://doi.org/10.1001/jama.2009.1811.

If needed, show the doctor the quote and ask that they refrain from unpleasant things to make matters worse, or from any care that would worsen the medical condition.

Please end the statement with "Thank you, Doctor."

Transition Process: From Adolescent to Adult Care

It's well known that patients and families love their pediatric and adolescent doctors but when they transition to adult care, they go through a significantly negative patient experience stemming in part from a negative engagement. This includes a dismissive attitude about their pain, and lack of human value, and being identified with derogatory terms, including negative labels such as drug seekers. There have been cases where patients with SCD choose to stay with their adolescent physician well through to their late twenties. I thought developing a personalized transition of care would hopefully put to rest negativity in obtaining healthcare in the adult world. For example, if my primary care physician thinks I need to see a cardiologist, he will give me a referral to someone that he knows and trusts. This should be no different for transition of care for patients with Sickle Cell disease.

Develop a transition process and protocols for adolescent transitioning to adult care.

Steps for transition care processes for adolescents and young adults with SCD to adult care

- The adolescent physician should identify and reach out to the adult physician that he or she believes would be an appropriate transition partner and schedule an appointment for transitioning young adult patients and family to be seen by the adult physician. The personalized transfer will result in better patient engagement and compassionate caring when the individual ages out of adolescence to adult care. The intent is for the new adult primary care physician to get to know the individual who is transitioning to adult care.
- In this current post-COVID and/or telehealth era, the initial conference and/or Zoom call with the adolescent, primary care

adult physician, patient, and family if the patient wants to include family members may be more appropriate. Care Managers should be on the call as well.
- Discuss medication and dosage required to relieve pain crisis.
- Coordinate care with an adult hematologist.
- Discuss comorbid conditions if applicable and recommendations for sub-specialists in those comorbid disease categories.
- Assess the mental needs of the individual, including depression screening and family therapy if needed

Patient Stories from Elmhurst

At Elmhurst Hospital, for me it was a journey, and at times it was a personal one. I will never forget the scared and frightened Chinese American mother at Elmhurst Hospital who came early every morning to the neonatal intensive care unit (NICU). Her newborn had cardiac surgery at Mount Sinai, the affiliate hospital, a week prior and now he needed to be transferred back to Mount Sinai Hospital for additional surgery.

I spoke with the NICU clinical team about her concerns regarding the need for a second surgery, and I was told they were waiting for her husband to arrive to explain the reason. I assumed he was parking the car and stated that he should be here shortly. The staff explained to me that they decided to wait for her husband since in the Chinese family the husband was the decision-maker. They were waiting until evening, when he came from work, to discuss their newborn's need for additional surgery. The concerns of the mother were totally ignored.

And so here was this mother in extreme anguish not knowing that the staff had made assumptions based on what they knew about the culture and were keeping information from her until the husband arrived from work. I truly felt her emotional and mental pain and fears, having been through a similar experience with my son when he required brain surgery at seventeen months old, as I tried to wipe away my tears as we sat and talked.

When I became aware of this action by the staff, I met with the clinical team and told them that "the Mommy Culture is front and center." It was a phrase that resonated with me at that moment, because collectively all mothers irrespective of culture, ethnicity, race, socioeconomic status, and country of origin have a unique maternal instinct and bond with our children at birth and throughout their entire life. Mothers experience pain when our babies are sick and hospitalized. I informed them that she was the mom, her name was on the birth certificate, and she was an American citizen. Equally important, she was extremely scared and in tremendous emotional pain and suffering for her baby. Being of Chinese descent did not mean they couldn't explain to her the need for the second surgery. They could explain to her, and then if she wished, let her tell them to wait for her husband. But to leave her stranded in anguish for hours was not the appropriate approach. It was not that the clinical team intended to harm, it was their perception that it was a culturally challenging decision.

In this instance, she had to know what was going on even if her husband was not around. The "mommy culture" provides the opportunity for the primary parent, in this case the mother, to have the influence, competence and control over their child's health or their own life circumstances. To me, this was a critical component of cultural sensitivity training. They needed to explain to her that nothing went wrong with the first surgery; but that it was that the cardiac surgery required two surgical procedures. After they spoke and explained the reason for the second surgery, the unimaginable burden was lifted, and she reached out and we hugged each other—a moment I will never forget, as it is embedded in my heart. Ultimately, I was glad to hear that the second surgery was successful.

Collaboration with the ED Director

The emergency department was the point of entry at both hospitals. Unlike private hospitals, there are extremely few direct inpatient admissions that do not go through the emergency room. The Care Management program was implemented first at Elmhurst and then at Queens.

Dr. Stuart Kessler, Medical Director of the ED at Elmhurst Hospital, was very supportive and a major collaborator with the implementation and success of the Care Management program in the emergency room. He educated me about the operation and the triage process based on severity of illness when an individual presents to the ED and introduced me and the care managers to the ED clinical team and explained their roles and responsibilities. Dr. Kessler and I had weekly scheduled meetings, and as a result I provided updates to the ED Care Management team. We also discussed our challenges and always received feedback and recommendations from Dr. Kessler.

Dr. Kessler also decided to assign Dr. Caryn Colombo, who sadly is no longer with us, to a lead role to provide guidance and education for the care managers. A significant role of the care managers in the ED was to coordinate care for complex patients who were being discharged from the ED, including ambulatory care follow-up appointments, homecare intervention when needed, and communication with the inpatient Bridge Team for patients who were admitted. We had weekly scheduled meetings with Dr. Colombo to discuss cases that were assigned to the care managers and their outcomes. The Care Management program in the ED that was supported by Dr. Kessler resulted in decreased visits to the ED for patients who were care managed. The ED Care managers also collaborated with the Bridge Team.

At Elmhurst, for example, one proud Hispanic dad with diabetes came to the emergency room every other day to check his blood sugar and was labeled noncompliant and a frequent flyer. From a Care Management perspective, it was not acceptable to use the word noncompliant or frequent flyer without asking WHY. The term noncompliant is generally used to refer to a patient who intentionally refuses to take a prescribed treatment or care plan and does not follow the recommendations that have been given by the doctor or care team.

He was assigned to the ED care manager, and when asked why he had come to the ED to check his blood sugar, he responded proudly by telling us that his son, who was a freshman in college in New Mexico, told him to stop taking the medication and to check his blood sugar at the emergency room as he lived only two blocks away.

When asked why his son told him to stop his medication, he said that his son had read an article that the medication killed two people in London, and he was not going to let his dad be the third. He stated so proudly, "My son knows what's best for me."

The Bridge Team met and discussed how best to transition the patient from recurrent ED visits to ambulatory care successfully. I remember that one of the care managers made a comment, "So we are supposed to take advice from an eighteen-year-old in New Mexico as to how we should provide care for his dad?"

I reminded the team of the patient's statement that his son knew what was best for him. My response was that there was no way we were going to solve the problem without including his son in the conversation about changing his recurrent ED visits and the staff's frustration with him as a "frequent flyer." We contacted his son and asked him to share the article that referenced the diabetic medication, Metformin, which was prescribed for his dad, but he was not able to find it. The team reassured him that he would be assigned to a primary care physician in ambulatory care, as well as a care manager who would be following up with him and his dad on a regular basis. We also told his dad that we were very proud of his son, and he teared up and hugged the care manager. The collaborative events resulted in significantly decreased visits to the ED, compliance with medication, and primary care appointments kept. Another stop-in-your-tracks teaching moment. Priceless!

I am so honored to know that the Bridge Team is still operational at Elmhurst Hospital, with additional staff inclusive of a pharmacist. The Sickle Cell Support Group is also still operational at Queens Hospital.

CHAPTER 4

Kings County Hospital– Merging of The African Diaspora

It was a difficult decision to leave my position as Associate Executive Director, Care Management, as my experience at Queens Health Network was amazing because of the interdepartmental and interdisciplinary collaboration, and particularly the positive results that were obtained that demonstrated sustainability and are still operational today. Prior to leaving, I received a lot of good wishes and compliments. I will share one here that was humbling.

> *Dear Dr. B,*
>
> *What is the patient not saying that we are not hearing? I learned this from you. It goes without saying that it was a great learning experience working with you. But to know you, your attitude toward people of all kinds, to your principles and beliefs, helped me grow personally and professionally. Congratulations and good luck in your new endeavor.*
>
> *Prajakta Vagal*

Why I chose to be Deputy Executive Director of Kings County Hospital

In August 2011, Mr. Antonio Martin, then CEO of NYC Health and Hospital, Kings County Hospital, invited me to Kings County to discuss possible opportunities. He wanted me to have a series of interviews, meaning I would be interviewed by senior management, and in addition, I was given the opportunity by Mr. Martin to interview senior management and anyone of my choosing, as well.

After meetings and several bi-directional interviews with several members of the staff, including Dr. Abba Agarwal, Chief Medical Officer, in September Mr. Martin offered me the position of Deputy Executive Director, Care/Case Management of Kings County Hospital, which at the time did not have a Care Management program.

I accepted the position because I was very interested in the uniqueness of Kings County Hospital's population. Approximately 95 percent of patients at NYC H+H/Kings County were of African ancestry, and most of them were English-speaking African Americans and Caribbean Americans with their second language being French/Creole. Interestingly, a substantial number of the Spanish-speaking population were from Panama. The top three Caribbean islands where patients originated, included Haiti, Jamaica, and Trinidad and Tobago. I thought it important to examine the migration stories of these populations to New York.

The majority of African Americans in New York City originally migrated from North and South Carolina. Just thirty-five years after the Emancipation Proclamation, African American communities had already begun to thrive. One community was the city of Wilmington, North Carolina, which thrived economically as they built churches, schools, and business until the massacre of 1898 by the Ku Klux Klan.

By 1900, significant portions of the African American population had begun migrating from North and South Carolina to New York (from 1876 to 1965) to escape the atrocities of the Ku Klux Klan, lynchings, and Jim Crow Laws.

Interestingly, the first involuntary journey for Afro Caribbean people to the US started when enslaved Barbadians were taken by the British to South Carolina during the seventeenth century. Most of the earliest Africans to arrive in what would become the United States were seasoned slaves, men, women, and children from the Caribbean.

Voluntary migration of Afro Caribbean people started at the turn of the twentieth century and the third wave, which consisted mostly of laborers and guest workers from the British West Indies, was fom 1930-1965. In terms of the Caribbean population, the top islands were Jamaica, Haiti, Guyana, Trinidad, and Tobago.

The Afro Caribbean population came to New York for a better life without experiencing the atrocities their African American counterparts had encountered and continue to live with. One group was part of a majority culture, the other was part of a minority culture. Over time in the United States, all became part of a minority culture; some more prepared than others to understand that they were no longer a part of the majority culture.

My Own Family Background

When you are part of a majority culture and you become part of a minority culture, as my family did when we came to America, that takes preparation, and as I stated earlier, some have more preparation than others. For my family, that transition took place over five years.

My dad migrated to America in 1957. This was during the Second Great Migration from the southern states and the Caribbean that began in 1940 and ended around 1970. Many Jamaicans were making that move at the time in pursuit of new economic opportunities, and the idea of doing so appealed to my father's entrepreneurial spirit. He settled in the Bronx across the Harlem River from Manhattan. I was five years old at the time. My mother completed her pharmacy degree and soon followed my dad to the US and left my siblings and me in the care of our amazing grandparents. We would visit Mom and Dad during the summer months, then we would return to Jamaica to continue our schooling. These vacation trips occurred each summer until I was ten years old, when we all migrated together to the United States for our new life. My parents lived then in a walkup apartment building without an elevator in the South Bronx.

My first experience with racism, which I did not understand, was when I was ten years old. I accompanied my younger brother downstairs as he saw children playing in front of our building through the window. They were boys playing tag with each other, and he asked them if he could join in. The response was, "If you want to play with us you have to scrub yourself white."

My brother and I had no clue what that meant. We didn't know they were referring to skin color, as where we grew up in Rockfort, Kingston, in Jamaica everyone on our block and in the neighborhood was Black, Chinese, or Indian, and we just knew we were all Jamaicans. I remember thinking that they were stupid and how do you scrub yourself White and for what purpose?

My father started out as a truck driver at a food and beverage distribution company, delivering to supermarkets in different communities throughout the Bronx. He was the only Black delivery man working for the company. If you were a White driver, you had somebody helping you. But because he was Black, he didn't. And if somebody stole from the truck while he was taking a delivery into the store, the cost was deducted from his paycheck.

My mother got a job as a bookkeeper. They weren't hiring Black people as pharmacists back then. In time, however, my parents ended up doing quite well in the Bronx. With their combined earnings, and with my mother as the bookkeeper handling the finances, they were eventually able to relocate from the South Bronx to the East Bronx, a much better neighborhood, bought a two-family home and acquired several rental properties.

I always wanted to be a doctor since I was a child. I am not sure why my relocation to America at ten years of age and growing up and experiencing life in the Bronx did not change my dream.

I graduated from James Monroe High School and was accepted to Boston University, where I graduated with a degree in biological science and subsequently went on to medical school at the University of Buffalo Jacob School of Medicine and Biological Science.

Appreciation of both African American and Caribbean History

In Jamaica, as well as other Caribbean islands, there was never a Rosa Parks moment. Rosa Parks was an African American civil rights icon because she refused to give up her seat on the bus to a White male in Montgomery, Alabama.

If you didn't get a seat on the bus in Jamaica or other Caribbean islands, it had 100 percent nothing to do with being Black. It was because you didn't have the money for the ticket, or because there simply wasn't an empty seat. The Caribbean population did not have to endure the atrocities of the Ku Klux Klan, lynching, and Jim Crow. In Jamaica we never talked about slavery. We just knew we were under British Colonial rule. And we never said we were Black; we were Jamaican irrespective of one's ethnicity. There were significant Indian and Chinese populations that came as indentured servants by the British. We all just merged into one culture, speaking English and Jamaican patois, and all identified as Jamaicans, we did not identify by ethnicity.

There is a historical relationship between Panama and the English-speaking Caribbean population, as the English-speaking Caribbean population under British colonial rule was sent to

Panama to build the Panama Canal. Panamanians were a large part of the Hispanic population at Kings County and were predominantly English-speaking, as well. Their names tended to be English and Spanish, e.g., Reinaldo Austin, Antonio Martin.

Here is a little bit of history about Kings County Hospital. It was founded in the East Flatbush neighborhood in Brooklyn, New York in 1830. It is affiliated with SUNY Downstate College of Medicine and is a designated Level 1 Trauma Center. Kings County Hospital has claimed many "firsts" in the field of medicine. It was the site for the first open heart surgery performed in New York State, invented the first hemodialysis machine, conducted the first studies of HIV infection, produced the first human images using magnetic resonance imaging (MRI), and was the first hospital in the US designated as a Level 1 Trauma Center.[14]

I had reached out to the Advisory Board, which is an organization that combines research, technology, and consulting to improve the performance of healthcare organizations, of which NYC H+H had membership. The question that I asked the Advisory Board was, "Can you identify any hospital across the nation where the hospital's population is predominantly Black, that improved the health of the population, the patient experience, and reduced cost using The Institute of Healthcare Improvement (IHI) Triple Aim concept?"[15]

I was told there was none. Currently, there is a Quadruple Aim,[16] which also includes provider satisfaction.

---

14 Kings County Hospital Center, Wikipedia Kings County Hospital Center History and Services (accessed May 2023) "Kings County Hospital Center." Wikipedia, January 31, 2024. https://en.wikipedia.org/wiki/Kings_County_Hospital_Center.
15 Triple Aim for Populations, Institute for Healthcare Improvement "Improvement Area: Triple Aim and Population Health." Institute for Healthcare Improvement. Accessed February 5, 2024. https://www.ihi.org/improvement-areas/triple-aim-population-health.
16 Derek Feeley, The Triple Aim or the Quadruple Aim? Four Points to Help Set your Strategy , Institute for Healthcare Improvement, November 2017 Feeley, Derek. "The Triple Aim or the Quadruple Aim? Four Points to Help Set Your Strategy." Institute for Healthcare Improvement, November 28, 2017. https://www.ihi.org/insights/triple-aim-or-quadruple-aim-four-points-help-set-your-strategy.

There was no doubt in my mind that NYC H+H, Kings County Hospital had the opportunity to be that amazing hospital that could accomplish being the first hospital with a predominantly Black population to meet the Triple Aim and could add another dimension to its amazing history.

Within a few weeks at Kings County, I visited various departments including surgery, medicine, behavioral health, pediatrics, intensive care units, ambulatory care, social work, nursing, utilization management, and the ED. I also attended several senior management meetings, community advisory boards, and "Break Through" meetings. Break Through is a part of the Lean Methodology used to develop and implement process improvement methodology to improve patient care in hospitals.

My role and responsibility were to implement a Care Management program and design a process to meet Project RED requirements that were mandated by NYC H+H, Central Office. Project RED (Re-Engineered Discharge) is a patient-centered approach to discharge planning and discharge education.

CHF 30-day Readmission Prevention Process and Results

Project RED was developed by the Agency for Healthcare Research and Quality (AHRQ). The goal was to decrease thirty-day readmission for patients with congestive heart failure (CHF). If a patient was readmitted within a thirty-day timeframe from the initial admission date, The Center for Medicare and Medicaid Services (CMS), which is a Federal agency within the Department of Health and Human Services that provides health coverage to more than 160 million Americans, would deny hospital payments for the second admission, unlike the historic precedent when CMS would pay for all readmissions.

Understanding the history and cultural norms of this predominantly English-speaking Black population had a major impact on the success of CHF task force results. When I designed and implemented the Care Management program, it went beyond discharge planning and education, which were the requirements of Project RED. The Chief Medical Officer of Kings County, Abha Agrawal, M.D., expressed to me that the CHF readmission rate was 30 percent. Kings County Hospital joined the Project RED mandate approximately nine months after all H+H hospitals.

The system's process began in 2011, and Kings County Hospital Center (KCHC) joined in 2012. We were able to decrease thirty-day readmission for CHF from 30 percent to 18.7 percent in two years. We accomplished this at times in a conventional manner and at other times in an unconventional manner.

Simply put, heart failure, sometimes known as CHF, occurs when your heart muscle doesn't pump blood as it should. Certain conditions such as narrowed arteries in your heart (coronary artery disease) or high blood pressure gradually leave your heart too weak or stiff to fill and pump efficiently. Not all conditions that lead to heart failure can be reversed, but treatments can improve the signs and symptoms of heart failure and help an individual live longer. Lifestyle changes—such as exercising, reducing sodium in your diet, managing stress, and losing weight—can improve your quality of life. One way to prevent heart failure is to prevent and control conditions that cause heart failure, such as coronary artery disease, high blood pressure, diabetes, or obesity.

Perception versus Reality Surveys

In remembering the perception versus the reality as to who the individuals with Sickle Cell were, I thought it would be helpful and informative to assess the perception versus reality of the patient population served by Kings County Hospital staff. If the perception were the same as reality, then designing and transforming a healthcare delivery system would have a higher degree of success. However, if the perception of the population served was not the reality, then the transformational techniques would be subject to failure. For example, if the perception of the population being insured is less than the reality, would that perception influence how the population would be perceived? Would it be positive or negative?

I felt it was crucial to design a staff survey that addressed the concept of perception versus reality of the predominantly African Diasporic populations served by Kings County Hospital. Most nationwide hospital surveys, including Hospital Consumer Assessment of Healthcare Providers and Systems (HCAHPS), aim to understand how patients feel about their hospital experience, the care they received, their opinion about the clinical team who treated their medical condition, and if they would recommend the hospital. To my knowledge, no required survey addresses the staff's feelings about the population served. From my perspective, how the staff feels about the population served can have a direct effect on patient care and HCAHPS scores—positive or negative.

I developed a staff survey for completion by the inpatient, ambulatory care, and emergency department staff to assess their perception of the patient population served. The objective was to compare their assumptions about the patient's socio-demographic information and related health statistics to what was accurate information or the reality. Below are some responses to the survey questions and the comparison with the reality:

Survey for hospital staff

Question	Perception	Reality
What percentage of the population have health insurance coverage?	Predominant Answer: 25 to 30 percent	75 percent of patients are insured
What percentage of the patient population is discharged to shelters?	Predominant Answer: 25 to 30 percent	3-5 percent of the population go to shelters
What percentage of the adult population is literate?	Predominant Answer: **meaning 35 percent literacy rate.** 65 percent illiterate	Literacy rate in the dominant population, which is Caribbean, was 90 percent, other than Haiti, which was 57 percent. Literacy rate for African Americans was 55 percent

On a personal note, I wondered if staff engagement with patients would be different if they realized that their assumptions did not align with the reality about the patient population served. I wondered whether knowledge of this reality would influence their behaviors, and as a result heighten patient value, improve patient engagement, and possibly result in better health outcomes, patient satisfaction, and lower costs. Improving the health of populations, increasing patient satisfaction, and reducing costs was the Triple Aim for healthcare improvement at that time.

Based on my research and understanding of the population served at Kings County, it was clear that a more engaging, nonjudgmental, empathetic, and cultural sensitivity patient engagement process had to be designed and implemented.

I implemented the Bridge Team concepts that I had developed in my previous position at Kings County with remarkable success. The interdisciplinary team was amazing and inclusive of nurse care and case managers, hospitalists, pharmacists, social workers, dietitians, rotating homecare services, clerical associates, and patients (if they were able to ambulate) at our morning meetings, along with the patients' families on the phone and a cardiologist as a consultant. The nurse care managers still practiced nursing, but nurse case managers were further removed from direct nursing care and became responsible for all communications with all health plans, including commercial, managed care, and union plans including long-term care and homecare services.

The team met every morning from 9-10 a.m. Monday through Friday on D4South, since the majority of patients with CHF were admitted to that unit. We discussed each individual patient, including reasons for admission, readmission, clinical condition, differentiated newly diagnosed CHF and previously diagnosed CHF, medications, labs, X-ray results, comorbid conditions, living arrangements, and follow-up appointments, including primary care and cardiology. There were unique deliverables that the team had to commit and adhere to that defined our transformation processes.

History Matters

When we reviewed the medical records, the words "noncompliant" and "nonadherent" were notable. What was also notable was the lack of a follow-up subjective reason for stating why an individual was noncompliant or nonadherent. The question "why" to understand the reason a patient didn't follow directions or did not follow the prescribed treatment regimen was rarely recorded. Why was it important for the team to commit to never using the word "noncompliant" without asking "Why?" For reference, if the clinical team did not know why an individual did not take his or her medication, why would that same medication that the patient didn't take be prescribed again? Why not further inquire about reasons for not being able to take the medication to figure out whether there were any negotiable options? The question is: Can clinical care be effective, and can we promote improved health outcomes, without further probing the simple and obvious "Why" question?

The "why" question was crucial because it could potentially eliminate conscious and unconscious Bias from the staff's perceptions and create an environment of empathy as opposed to judgmental attitudes from the clinical teams. The practice of not further inquiring and asking "Why," can result in making adverse and biased decisions—one of the potential contributors to poorer health outcomes, particularly for African Americans.

I have conducted multiple presentations at conferences in my current role as President, Mauvareen Beverley, M.D. PLLC, Patient Engagement and Cultural Competence Specialist, where attendees include clinicians, nurses, social workers, administrative staff, and public health professionals from across the country and from diverse health systems and organizations. During these presentations, I would routinely ask the question, "How many times have you used or heard the word noncompliant to describe patients?"

The overwhelming response would usually be 100 percent. When I raised the second question, "How many times have you seen written in the medical records or heard the reason why when noncompliant or nonadherent is used," maybe one or two attendees raised their hands.

The overwhelming response to the "Why" question when I began these talks was that there was unanimous agreement about the absence of the "Why" when the word noncompliance was used when describing a patient's lack of compliance with medications, lifestyle changes, referrals, etc. Now we use the less toxic word nonadherence to substitute for noncompliance. Interestingly, the "Why" question is still not part of the nonadherence conversation.

Most medical providers, including medical students, interns, residents, and attending physicians are trained to always ask "Why" when it comes to diagnosing a condition. Why does the patient have a fever, abdominal pain, elevated white count, slurred speech, chest pain, etc.? However, when it comes to a patient not complying with instructions or not taking medications, the "Why" question is not usually a requirement. It also has been documented that negative terminology in medical records are written two to three times more often in describing African Americans than Whites. As a result, I would venture to say that the "Why" question is less applicable to African American patients.

Train Driver Patient Story: Noncompliant without the "Why" Question

This is a typical admitting statement:

"60 y/o African American male recently diagnosed two weeks ago for new onset Congestive Heart Failure (CHF) returns to the emergency room and is readmitted for heart failure decompensated due to noncompliance with medications."

In any hospital, when this description of a patient assigned to a unit on the inpatient service is used, they experience a judgmental attitude and lack of caring because their decompensated medical condition will be considered the patient's own fault. A care manager on our team met with the patient and asked why he didn't take his medication. He was insistent that he could not take the Lasix, which he referred to as a "water pill" which is a common term that's used by doctors and patients.

He was then asked why he couldn't take the water pill. He responded: "I can't take the water pill because I drive the number six train." His reason was because he operated the New York City number six subway train as an engine driver. The diuretic that he had been given to treat fluid retention (edema) and swelling that is caused by CHF resulted in increased urination. We pulled up his medical record to see what was recorded in his social history. Interestingly, on this admission form, he was described as unemployed. I embraced the possibility that when he was first admitted because of the severity of his illness, his social history was not a priority. He explained that his work shift was from 11 p.m. to 11 a.m. He was then asked what he did when he got home, and he stated that he ran errands, had breakfast, took some of his medications, and then he would take a nap and take his water pill after dinner when he was not on his shift.

The cardiologist was consulted and told him to take the Lasix after breakfast and cautioned him that it may wake him up from sleep, but that it would be much earlier in the day as opposed to closer to his night work schedule. In addition, we would provide a cubicle that he could use in a private space when the train stopped at a station. His response was, "If I knew I had to choose between peeing and breathing, I would have chosen breathing."

It was clearly an educational and memorable moment for me and the team. It's possible that without our team engaging the patient in a nonjudgmental, caring manner, asking "Why," and valuing him as a human being, he may have died prematurely—and his death could possibly have been attributed to noncompliance with medications at the mortality report. It is also a learning curve for us to recognize the difficulty when a patient must make a choice between their health and their employment.

The irony is that on some occasions, it would be that same medication—that the records stated the patient was noncompliant with *and did not ask why*— that would be refilled for the patient when discharged to home. This is not unique to Kings County Hospital. There was a shared mindset and buy-in concerning language that was off-limits. It was important for hospital staff to understand that labels and bias were harmful to patients. Labels of drug seekers, noncompliant, frequent flyers, and other stereotypes often led to biased care and adverse outcomes. In addition to not using "noncompliant" without asking "Why" and eliminating the use of the term frequent flyers, patients were given the benefit of the doubt. This approach helped to create a culture of empathy as opposed to judgmental behavior.

I believe if noncompliant is written in a patient's medical record two or three times, then the negative descriptor results in disregard for the health and well-being of the patient. As a result, patient engagement is reduced to a minimum, and that individual now has to maneuver themselves through the complicated health system. I am also of the belief that health systems turn "noncompliant patients" into another negative terminology, "Frequent Flyers," because they end up in the emergency room or being readmitted for care. This is a domino effect, since they must navigate their way through the complex health system that has judgmental attitudes and a lack of empathy. Just a thought.

There needs to be a shared mindset and buy-in by the health system concerning language that is off-limits. In addition to not using "noncompliant/nonadherent" without asking "Why" and eliminating the use of the term "frequent flyers," giving the patients the benefit of the doubt, and creating a culture of empathy as opposed to judgmental behavior is an important requirement for achieving health equity.

The quote below is a powerful statement that exposes and exemplifies honesty related to systemic or institutional inequities and the challenging issues that healthcare professionals should and must address is applicable in this context as well.

"Difficult patients are not just born, they are, in part, created by their passage through the medical system. Not only has this system failed to cure, but it may also have done unpleasant things to make matters worse."—Dr. William T. Zempsky

Who is the Individual?

On morning rounds with the clinical team that was responsible for patient care, the readmission prevention team would sometimes join the rounds, including myself.

For example, the clinical team rounded on two patients in a room with two beds for double occupancy. The first patient was in his bed closest to the door and the second patient was in his bed closest to the window. Both patients were awake and alert and were willing to participate by answering questions.

The clinical team spoke with and examined the patient closest to the entrance with closed curtains, then went to see the patient by the window. After examining and assessing the patient, the team asked, "Do you have any questions?"

The patient's response was what I refer to as a stop-in-your-tracks moment." He pointed to the patient in the other bed and said, "I am not him and he is not me, we don't know each other. You know neither one of us, but you are telling us the same thing."

Needless to say, his response was not anticipated and there was a period of silence.

I stepped in and apologized to him and told him that in the event we gave him the idea that both individuals were interchangeable, we were deeply sorry. I explained that the reason the conversation was similar is that most of the patients on this unit have the same medical condition; then I asked if the treatment and medications he had received made him feel better. He said that they had. I could not help but wonder if there had not been a response to his statement and concerns, would he have believed his diagnosis and followed our directions or would he have signed out against medical advice (AMA)? I am happy to report that he did neither. Interestingly, as we left the room and were having a conversation in the hall, one of the interns stated that he was surprised that the patient understood the word "interchangeable." This was another example of perception versus reality of the individual's level of intelligence and who he was.

Understanding the individual and their intellectual analysis in a nonjudgmental manner was a key teaching moment. All individuals, irrespective of insurance access or status, whether limited or lacking thereof, education level, occupation, socioeconomic status, beliefs, race, or gender have their own personal assessment of their medical problems and how the hospital staff sees them.

Role of Social History

Another key component to knowing the individual patient is how they are described in social history. An individual's social history is a major requirement in medical school training. Social history must include whether the patient is married, single, separated, or divorced; their living arrangements; their employment status (for example: retired postal worker or unemployed); along with their level of education, primary language, and religion. However, in most circumstances, the social history just states: nondrinker, nonsmoker, or no toxic substance. Could one imagine an elderly Black patient who has been in church since birth, is only described in her social history in terms of being a nondrinker/nonsmoker or no toxic substance instead of her faith and spirituality, which is more meaningful? The bar for understanding the individual has become exceptionally low. A social history should provide a sense of the patient's background—it gives a holistic picture of the individual. Limiting social history to a smoking or drinking status does not provide a holistic picture of their socioeconomic background or culture, preferences, or values. It is not surprising that the need for patient engagement, empathy, and compassion has taken a lower priority given that most often, social history is limited to a smoking or drinking status. Again, this description of an individual and their social history in the electronic health records is not unique to Kings County Hospital. In my opinion, it is present across the country. It made me reflect on my medical training once again at Harlem Hospital where a comprehensive social history was the norm.

Patient Fears: A Moving and Riveting Example of the Relationship between Noncompliance, Patient, and Family Fears.

Interestingly, when I reviewed the medical literature as it relates to patient fears, I found that there is not much information to be found. In terms of noncompliance, I do believe that a patient's fears could possibly be a major contributing factor.

For example, one patient was experiencing worsening renal failure and persistently refused hemodialysis. "Noncompliant" was all over this person's inpatient and outpatient medical records documentation. In the team discussion, I asked if anyone had spoken with his wife? The answer was no. The only person that would be able to convince him, in my opinion, would be his wife. We scheduled a meeting with his wife, and I explained the seriousness of his condition as a life-and-death circumstance. I asked why her husband did not want the dialysis treatment for his life-threatening condition and if she could convince him to do so? Much to my surprise, she said, "I don't think I want to convince him to do so."

I asked her to tell me why. She expressed in a scared, sad, and fearful way that she would not be able to live with herself if she convinced him. The pain and suffering she was experiencing were very visible and hit me in the gut. I had to ask the "why" question once again.

She went on to explain that their neighbor had gone on dialysis and two weeks later he died. It was humbling. Based on what she shared, I wonder if we as healthcare professionals would rush to convince our loved one to go on dialysis based on her experience? It was an emotional moment for me, and I was committed to helping her and her husband to agree to dialysis and enable her to live with herself without the irreparable guilt she thought she would have to endure.

I reached out to the nephrologist, who met with the patient and his wife. He explained that he couldn't say why their neighbor had died; that it could have been due to end-stage kidney disease, or he could have had a heart attack, a blood clot to the lungs, or something else. He realized that they needed hand-holding and recognized the need for him to tamp down their fears and reassure them that if the patient were to accept dialysis, he would be right there with them for the first week, and if needed thereafter. The patient accepted dialysis and as a result did much better.

This example was patient engagement, compassion, and empathy at its best. As a result, fear factor conversations became front and center during team meetings.

Crossroads Between Fears and What's Important to the Individual

One very contentious and angry African American male patient was quite problematic in the sense that he would yell and scream whether he was answering or asking a question. The nurses had had it with him, and understandably so. There was something about this individual that I wanted to know more about because of his contentious anger when asked simple questions. I went to see him and introduced myself, and he said in a loud and angry voice, "What do you want?"

I asked in a quiet and calm voice, "Will you be willing to share with me what's important to you?"

His demeanor and body language changed, and he had tears in his eyes as opposed to anger. He answered sadly and in no uncertain terms, "Attending my granddaughter's wedding!"

I asked next if he was concerned that he would not be able to attend? He looked down at the floor with tears in his eyes and answered in a softer, emotional, and scared voice, "Yes, I am afraid I will not make it to November for her wedding."

If memory serves me correctly, it was June or July at that time, and I reassured him in no uncertain terms that we recognized what was important to him and would collaborate with him in meeting his goal of attending his granddaughter's wedding.

We made sure that he had a cardiology appointment within a week post-discharge and a follow-up primary care physician (PCP) office visit after two weeks. The plan also included medication pickup (including a pill box, which he did not have), and homecare interventions. The care manager checked in with him weekly and had phone calls with homecare and communication with his cardiologist and primary care physician. He was not readmitted, and over the course of four months, we got to know the individual, pacify his fears, and learn what was important to him and where he was in the acceptance of his disease. He called us in November to let us know that he was so happy and thankful for our efforts and that his son told him he would be walking his granddaughter down the aisle at her wedding. The team was emotional. We were so happy for him. After he hung up, one team member asked in a funny and sarcastic way if we were invited to the wedding? NO! We all happily laughed and shared tissues.

The takeaway from that case is that if you have never lay in a hospital bed as a patient, it's difficult to understand the trauma, the fears about a potentially life-threatening condition that may change one's personality, and that coming to grips and defining what's important in life is now a priority.

I thought it important to design a survey to look at the perception versus reality about why patients don't take their medications. The survey was given to doctors, nurses, social workers, case managers who worked with inpatients and in the ED, and patients with CHF.

As I previously stated, congestive heart failure tends to be diagnosed in the elderly population, and our cohort of patients was no different even though we had a few patients under forty and one twenty-three-year-old patient whose story you will read in the next chapter.

What drove a lot of our passion and innovative thought processes were directly related to the patient voices, and there was a recognition that they were in our hospital beds and not in our history books once we heard their survival stories against all odds.

Had we not enhanced the patient value, expanded the social history to reflect the individual, approached patient engagement from the actual reality versus the perception, and eliminated negative terminology and the use of the term noncompliant without asking "Why," we would not have had the privilege, honor, and trust to improve their health outcomes by creating empathetic and nonjudgmental conversations that created a comfortable environment for the individual patient to tell their stories.

What I realized was that some of the elderly African Americans spoke in codes, e.g., "My family picked cotton on a plantation that was not ours."

Another major irony in the age of patient experience and cultural competence in the delivery of healthcare, is that the English-speaking population is not part of the cultural competence conversation, and as a result, may contribute to health disparities for African and Caribbean Americans along with the most vulnerable subset, the elderly African Americans.

The role of religion in this population, along with their tenacity, independence, and honesty, was not only humbling but inspirational.

Patient Voices:
They are in our Hospital Beds and Not in the History Books

A ninety-three-year-old African American female originally from South Carolina who had seven brothers stated, "My family picked cotton on a plantation that was not ours. We had to get up at the crack of dawn and pick 300 to 500 pounds of cotton a day and then I had to walk ten miles to a segregated school."

I was thinking that in today's world, we can't even walk five blocks without calling an Uber.

Question: How could you walk ten miles to school?
Answer: If you wanted an education, you had to walk. (I will never

forget the look on her face and her body language, as if to say, "What part of this don't you get, stupid?") I further asked, "Did you have to walk back home?" She stated that her principal took her home on a horse drawn carriage as they had to get back before dark as a result of the Ku Klux Klan. I asked how old she was when that occurred, and she responded that she had been ten years old.

She completed primary, junior high, and high school, then attended Voorhees College, but she stated, "I did not get in until the second semester."

Sixty years later, she was still upset with herself for not being accepted on her first try. She came to New York in 1942 at the age of twenty-five, married in 1948, and had two sons. They were the first two of five Black students to integrate into Stuyvesant High School. Her first son graduated from Columbia University and became a mechanical engineer. Her second son graduated from Stanford University and became an electrical engineer.

She graduated from city college and later became a registered nutritionist. She worked at a hospital in Brooklyn until she retired in the 1980s. When asked what her salary was at retirement, she said, "Two hundred dollars per week but others made more."

She was a Baptist. Her statement that "others made more" read between the coded lines.

Her tenacity, independence, and her survival against all odds were inspirational to say the least.

I also met an eighty-three-year-old Guyanese patient who said that her parents were slaves. I asked her to tell me more. She said, "My dad was on the tobacco plantation and my mom on the sugar plantation."

The plantations that they worked on and what the African slaves were forced to do was a matter of where the slave ships landed.

A seventy-two-year-old Trinidadian female was asked, ``How can I help?"

She stated in no uncertain terms, "You want to help me, get me out of this bed. Laying in this bed makes me lazy. I am used to moving around and doing things. Can you do that?"

When asked who took care of her, she said, "I take care of myself. I do my own shopping and my laundry."

When the nurse brought one eighty-four-year-old Guyanese female four medications and offered her water to take her meds, she stated, "I don't want your water; I have to eat then take one pill; eat again then take the rest the same way. By the way, is there Lasix in the cup? I don't want it; I was in the bathroom twelve times yesterday."

One eighty-four-year-old African American female originally from South Carolina said, "My parents were a step away from slavery and my grandparents were slaves."

It was humbling.

A seventy-six-year-old African American repeatedly told nurses, doctors, and social workers, "It's in God's hands" when discussions arose about what she needed to do to improve her health outcomes.

The clinical team took her responses to mean that she didn't want to take responsibility for her own health and blamed her circumstances on God. In meeting with the clinical team, I raised the possibility that she genuinely believed that her health condition is in God's hands.

At her bedside, my team and I told the patient that she was correct in her belief that her health was in God's hands. However, I also asked her if she would allow us to help God in improving her health as it's important for us to please God as well.

Her response: "Sister, shall we pray?" We all joined hands and prayed with her. Our conversation ended with AMEN, and as a result, we were able to earn her trust and better collaborate with her to improve her heart-related health outcomes.

An eighty-four-year-old Jamaican patient with heart failure was brought to the hospital by her children and grandchildren because she refused to take her medicines. When asked why she did not take her medications, she stated, "All the medications make me confused. I am in the bathroom all day because of the water pill, and I can't eat a morsel of anything I like. So, what's the point?"

Her statement echoes the importance of quality of life irrespective of age.

One seventy-eight-year-old African American female originally from South Carolina who was dissatisfied with her hospital experience stated, "I picked cotton in the South, and I paid my dues. I don't deserve to be treated this way."

We changed her doctor and gave her a geriatrician, gave her earlier appointments, had follow-up phone calls with her, and deeply apologized to her for her experience. I went to see her in ambulatory care for her first appointment with her geriatrician and asked about her experience.

I am happy to say she was appreciative and satisfied with the care she received. In her next statement she said, "Dr. Beverley, all I want when I come to a hospital is for everyone to be nice to me."

Her desire was simple, and I took that as a learning moment to educate the team. The takeaway was that individuals become combative in healthcare settings when their fears are not addressed; they don't feel respected, their dignity is compromised, and compassionate care was not an option given.

Conversation with a ninety-four-year-old African American male from Mississippi

I said to myself humorously, "Mississippi, you are supposed to be from the Carolinas; you are throwing my metrics off. Shouldn't you be in Chicago somewhere?"

On a more serious note, I asked the question, "When did you come to New York?"

He answered in the 1940s. I asked him what kind of work he did. "I was a Pullman porter on the train and my name was George." He raised his hands in the air and said, "George do this, George do that."

There was no identity; he, like all the other Pullman porters, was just called George. I told him, "You know your name isn't George, right? Thank you for being who you are; if it weren't for individuals like you, I wouldn't be here today. Please tell me, how can I help you?"

After meeting with this remarkable human being who endured, on a daily basis, a lack of individuality, dignity, and respect while carrying the weight of a people, I had what I described as my emotional stop-in-your-tracks breakdown moment.

I went to the team and said, "If they want to spend the rest of their lives on the beach, make it happen."

I was brought back to reality when the case manager said, "Dr. B, health plans don't pay for time on the beach."

I was back on track and deeply passionate about improving the health, recognition, and value of this population.

Pullman porters were men hired to work on the railroads as porters on sleeping cars. Starting shortly after the American Civil War, George Pullman sought out former slaves to work on his sleeper cars. Pullman porters served American railroads for one hundred years, from the late 1860s until late in the twentieth century. Pullman porters, who were largely Black, are widely credited with contributing to the development of the Black middle class in America. Under the leadership of A. Philip Randolph, Pullman porters formed the first all-Black union, the Brotherhood of Sleeping Car Porters, in 1925, which was instrumental as the first African American labor union to sign a collective bargaining agreement with a major US corporation[17].

When one eighty-nine-year-old Jamaican female with a diagnosis of dementia was asked where she was, she said, "Brookdale hospital."

---

17 Pullman Porter Wikipedia https://en.wikipedia.org/wiki/Pullman_porter#:~:text=Pullman%20porters%20were%20men%20hired,work%20on%20his%20sleeper%20cars. Assessed Feb 2023 "Pullman Porter." Wikipedia, January 5, 2024. https://en.wikipedia.org/wiki/Pullman_porter.

I told her that she was in Kings County, and she said, "Oh, yes." I thought that since that was during the Obama presidency, and she was Black, she may know who the President of the United States was. If not, there may be an element of dementia. So, I asked her who the president of the United States was, and she answered, "He has a funny name that I won't remember, but he has a very lovely wife and she's always with the older daughter and he is always with the younger one."

I told her that his name is Barack Obama. She said, "Yes, but I won't remember his name, but I do know he is African American."

The election of the first Black president of the United States superseded her dementia.

If we acknowledge our patients' history, we would know that some of our patients may have been part of the Civil Rights movement. Some of our patients may have suffered a level of atrocity more than we can ever imagine. It's important to recognize that access to care for some of our elderly Black patients had nothing to do with simply getting an appointment. History prevented them from getting care. Trust in the healthcare system is still a matter of concern for some (e.g., The USPHS Syphilis Study at Tuskegee).

Have a conversation; hear their story so that all of us share the same mindset in the belief that when any Black elderly individual leaves this Earth, it will be on their own terms and not because we as healthcare professionals chose not to recognize their historical and individual value to our institution, the country, and their families.

Some of our patients may have sacrificed their dignity for the betterment of a generation.

I recall a statement President Obama made in his 2008 "Speech on Race" when he stated, "I married a Black American woman who carries within her the blood of slaves and slaveowners—an inheritance we pass on to our two precious daughters." A timely recognition of our past.

For reference, when a Holocaust survivor gets admitted to a hospital in the United States, the hospital culture is to roll out the red carpet.

The Board of Directors, the Chief Executive Officer (CEO), the Rabbi, and the Chief Medical Officer (CMO) will visit the patients, and so they should as a result of the horrendous and horrific circumstances that they endured. When an African American elderly patient who fled the South because of the atrocities of the Ku Klux Klan, lynchings, Jim Crow, and segregation, there is no red carpet rolled out even though the atrocity happened right here in the US! It is an opportunity to learn and put into practice, the red carpet roll-out for all atrocity survivors and recognize that the role of religion in both groups was pivotal to their survival.

In March 1966, Martin Luther King Jr. delivered a speech at a convention of the Medical Committee for Human Rights. He said, "Of all the forms of inequality, injustice in healthcare is the most shocking and inhumane." At the time, Dr. King was conducting direct action to bring hold-out hospitals in line with the legal desegregation requirements of the Civil Rights Act passed one year earlier.

Because of our amazing results with CHF thirty-day readmission decrease, The Harlem Reunion event that was held at Harlem Hospital in 2017 to honor Dr. Gerald Thompson included a conference on the elderly African American population, with the majority of the speakers in various specialties who trained at Harlem Hospital. Most notably, the Keynote Speaker, Dr. Mary Bassett, then New York City Commissioner of Health and Dr. Nilsa Gutierrez, then Chief Medical Officer, Region DHHS Centers for Medicare & Medicaid Services Region 2.

Being at Kings County Hospital in my position of Deputy Executive Director, Care/Case Management was and still is an incredible and educational experience. I have learned so much from the staff there and from listening to the voices of the individuals who were hospitalized and lying in their beds with a potentially life-threatening illness; hearing their stories and concerns, recognizing patient fears, understanding what's important to the individual, and noting the time it takes in some instances for the patient's acceptance of the disease. On a personal note, I will share an unforgettable moment that a member of the team told me: "Dr. B, I was speaking to a nurse who repeatedly described a patient as noncompliant. She interrupted her co-worker and told her to go back to the patient and ask him "Why?"

It was an "each one, teach one" moment, and was very encouraging to see that my efforts were making a difference in how the patients were treated.

When there is recognition that change is needed in health systems institutional culture, and if done in a professional, compassionate, and nonjudgmental manner with staff and patient input, it has the potential for success and sustainability going forward.

I was asked if the team was stressed out about obtaining the results over the course of time. The answer when I asked the team was an unequivocal "No!"

As one team member stated, "We had a change in mindset about how we communicated with our patients, and we were on a mission to improve their health outcomes. In addition, we had fun and a great time."

CHAPTER 5

Medications and Adherence

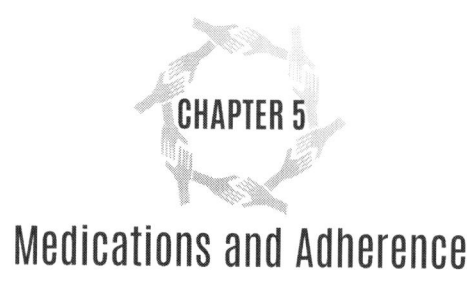

Do No Harm

After graduating medical school all physicians take the Hippocratic Oath "Do No Harm." To make an accurate diagnosis, the "Why" question is a major contributing factor. For example, why does the patient have a fever? Why the abdominal pain? Why the severe headache? Why the lab results? Why, Why, Why? However, when it comes to using the words noncompliant/nonadherent, why is there not a similar interest in knowing the reason why someone didn't follow directions?

Question: Why don't patients take their medications?
The answer from most staff was—"COST."

The answer from most patients was—"We think we are taking too many medications."

Not one patient mentioned cost. The average patient with heart failure with comorbid medical conditions was taking on average seven medications three times per day. Based on the patient response, the pharmacist on the team reviewed all patient medications and was able to eliminate and/or combine medications from seven to five medications per day. There is no doubt in my mind that adjusting and combining some of the medications contributed to the decrease in readmissions.

It's interesting to note that during a presentation with clinical teams, I asked the question, "How many of you are taking medications?" About fifteen attendees raised their hands. My next question asked how many were taking seven, six, five, four, three, two, or one type(s) of medication? No one was on four or more medications. Only three responded that they were on three medications, and one responded that he was on one medication that was an antibiotic that required him to take it twice per day. I asked him, "Are you compliant with your medication that you should take twice per day?"

He said, "No."

I asked him the "Why" question, and he said sometimes he forgot and sometimes it was based on his shift schedule. My response was, "So you are noncompliant with one medication and patients are taking on average five to seven medications, and we refer to them as noncompliant. It's an opportunity for us to understand what it must be like for a patient to comply with multiple medications."

He responded, "I totally understand now and will have a different conversation with patients, including the why question, and not be judgmental going forward."

Care Management Patient Information Tool (PIT)

I implemented the Care Management patient information tool to enhance communication, help patients stay engaged and involved in their medical decisions, and identify any needs and potential concerns. (See resources section for more information.)

We collected survey data from 445 patients with heart failure who responded to the tool. We identified the top three concerns of the patients, which included an expressed need or whether they would, (1) have results of laboratory and X-ray or imaging results in a timely manner, (2) be kept abreast of their medical condition and diagnosis, and (3) have homecare available upon discharge to their home.

Are patients really any different from us, who we are as professional healthcare providers? If we or our loved one were hospitalized, and given the PIT, wouldn't our top three concerns be the same or similar?

Unforeseen Circumstance: Lack of Pill Box

Most patients who are on several medications have difficulty managing their regimen, especially when there are inadequate dosage instructions upon discharge, changes in regimen or challenges with reconciling with new medications. Sometimes there are discrepancies between the regimen that was prescribed and what a patient thinks they should be taking. A pill box can be an asset to patients on multiple medications and regimens to help them organize their pills.

"Lack of Pill Box" was applicable to the majority of the cohort of patients prescribed multiple medications.

The fact that individual patients with CHF diagnosis are taking on average seven medications three times per day and did not have a pill box was alarming. This was because slight errors in how medications were taken at home could lead to unnecessary harm, disease progression, and eventual premature death. It was important to have a conversation about how one should take their medications to minimize discrepancies in the prescribed regimen and improve medication safety and health outcomes after discharge. This is also an opportunity to understand the individual's routine, to adjust the medication regimen accordingly. As a result of this conversation, staff can gain a greater understanding of the patient's knowledge of their regimen and do a better job of educating them if there are gaps in their understanding, as opposed to not getting the individual's input but only providing discharge planning directions based on protocol.

Another "Stop-in-Your-Tracks Moment"

One patient was asked, "Tell us how you take your medications on a daily basis?" Much to my surprise, he took a bottle out of his bag which held at least forty pills in multiple different sizes and colors.

He went on to explain that he took the white ones in the morning, the pink ones in the afternoon, and the different shaped white ones in the evening. When asked about whether he had a pill box, he was not aware of what that was.

It was at this moment that we implemented a "must ask" question: "Do you have a pillbox?"

Much to our surprise, we found out that approximately 50 percent of the admitted CHF patients did not have a pill box. A mandatory protocol was developed for all homecare services to provide and set up the pill box and provide instructions and education to patients and families referred free of charge.

Some solutions are as simple as they are complex. I would assume making sure everyone having a pill box had a major impact on decreasing readmissions.

The lack of a pill box was what I described as an "Unforeseen Circumstance."

Gemba Walk in a Patient's Home

What is a Gemba Walk? A Gemba walk is an important technique used by those interested in continuous improvement. The goal of the Gemba walk is to learn more about how processes are performed and to notice potential improvement opportunities.

What happens during a Gemba Walk? A supervisor, manager, or other leader goes to the place where work is done to get a deeper insight as to how processes are being performed and to spot potential opportunities for improvement.

During our interdisciplinary team morning meetings, a topic that was constantly discussed was the need for medication reconciliation. After a team discussion including pharmacist Miriam Klein, there was agreement that the most accurate medication reconciliation would be in the patient's home.

QUESTION: A First
Can we do a Gemba Walk in a selected patient's home?

ANSWER: YES
KCHC Leadership gave permission for Miriam Klein, the pharmacist, to do a Gemba Walk in a patient's home.

It was a bold initiative whose purpose was twofold: To do the ultimate medication reconciliation with the belief that the difference in outcomes is made in the patient's home and providing meaningful data to develop necessary protocol that will positively impact medication reconciliation, patient safety, and avoid readmission.

Tamor Daley, my secretary who scheduled and coordinated all my meetings and presentations, arranged transportation for Miriam to go to a patient's home, had the driver wait, then after the Gemba Walk drove Miriam back to KCHC.

Medication Issues identified in the Home

Some of Dr. Klein's findings in the home of a patient with congestive heart failure, diabetes, hypertension, and angina were as follows:

Medication	Issues
Furosemide (water pill)	Furosemide 40 mg twice a day was not filled by the community pharmacy as the time frame was not met for refill. Pharmacy did not note change—dosage changed from 40 mg to 20mg
Enalapril	Homecare RN did not have Enalapril on their medication list. Patient hand-wrote the medication's name.
Isosorbide Dinitrate	Not filled by pharmacy—time frame was not met. Patient had misplaced medication.
Herbal Medicine Concerns	Patient was taking garlic daily; he was not aware that it could decrease his blood sugar.
Other	Medications at home from his community PCP and KCHC were all in the same bottle.

Corrective Action Steps

- Educate homecare nurses to contact pharmacies regarding medication not filled in case of a change in dosage.
- Provide and set up pill boxes as well as educate the family and patient.

KCHC Pilot Intervention: A Collaboration with a Homecare Agency

Based on the results of the pharmacist's Gemba Walk in a patient's home, I decided to collaborate with a homecare agency to do a pilot program for medication reconciliation. Whenever a homecare nurse went to visit a patient's home, they were required to identify medications in the home along with learning who the prescriber was. Miriam Klein and the homecare pharmacist oversaw the pilot program.

There were sixty home visits in that initial pilot program. We found out that 28 percent of the medications being taken by the patient in the home were different from what was on record at Kings County. For example, KCHC had prescribed medication to accurately treat a patient for heart failure; however, the community physician had prescribed medication for treating asthma.

HOMECARE PROTOCOL

We created a personalized CHF discharge folder for each CHF patient. It included diagnosis, lab and X-ray results, medication list, medication instructions, follow-up appointments, homecare services, the PIT tool, and the Care Management department number to call if there were questions.

Checklist	Instructions
	Verify medication list that is in the patient's personalized CHF discharge folder. Explain the folder.
	Check and record all medications in the home, including herbal and over-the-counter medications.
	Complete and sign the medication reconciliation form and email Ms. Youseline Champagne, Associate Director of Care Management, within twenty-four hours of a home visit.
	If there was a significant discrepancy, the visiting nurse had to contact Ms. Champagne on the same day.
	Make sure patients have picked up all medications, and if not, state the reason why.
	Provide pillbox and set up medications and educate patients and families about how to set up the pill box with their medications.
	Educate patients and families about medications, including side effects of medications versus symptoms of disease.
	Verify use of herbal medicines and address patient's herbal concerns. For example, a patient was taking garlic daily and he was not aware that it could decrease his blood sugar.
	Provide a report to be presented at Friday's CHF pilot meeting.

Homecare nurses had to submit the medication forms that were given to them and fax them to the homecare agency, pharmacists, Miriam Klein, and Ms. Champagne.

Miriam Klein and I presented "Reducing Readmissions: CHF Pilot Team and a Gemba Walk in a Patient's Home" at The National Patient Safety Foundation's Fifteenth Annual Patient Safety Congress in New Orleans, Louisiana in May 2013.

CHAPTER 6

Two Illuminating Patient Stories

Ryan's Story

I am including my son's story in this book because his story made me realize the importance of a physician's caring, competence, and empathy for their patients—all important traits which helped me through the scariest time in my life. As I discussed earlier in Chapter Three, about the story of the Chinese American mom, I truly felt the pain and suffering she was going through of not knowing why her newborn needed another surgery. One does not have to experience what I went through to empathize with others, but hopefully it will shed light on the needed action to take, resulting in progress toward achieving health equity when each human being is valued.

I thought I would share my personal story about my favorite second-born son. As I stated earlier, many of us physicians have never been hospitalized, and those of us who have ever been hospitalized tend to be female physicians giving birth. Being a physician and a mom, I too was hospitalized for the births of my three sons. However, I never thought that I would experience the hospitalization of my son for brain surgery at seventeen months old. I was also hospitalized, as I spent every day, every hour, every second with him.

I always refer to my children as my favorite first-born, my favorite second-born, and my favorite third-born. Ryan is my favorite second-born. At birth he weighed ten pounds two ounces born via C-section, had no health issues, and was developing as scheduled, and in some cases quicker than expected. He walked at ten months and talked around the same time. There is a moment in one's life as a mother that you will remember for the rest of your life. I am no different.

When he was seventeen months old, I placed him in his crib, and he fell asleep. A little later I heard him moving around in his crib. I remember going over to him and smiling and was about to say, "What are you doing?"

To my shock, Ryan, my favorite second-born, was having a generalized seizure with a right focal component (seizure that primarily affects the right side of the brain). I cannot remember a time in my life that I was so frightened. I turned him on his side to prevent choking and called my husband in a panic. We both supported him on his side until the seizure was resolved; it seemed like an eternity and not a few minutes. He was afebrile (no fever), and the cause of the seizure was brain cancer—that was my deepest fear.

I immediately called Dr. Carolyn Britton, Attending Neurologist at Columbia Presbyterian Medical Center (CPMC) who had trained at Harlem Hospital, and she immediately made arrangements for Ryan to see the pediatric neurologist at CPMC. I was then referred to the Children's Hospital of Philadelphia, and subsequently to Dr. Epstein (RIP), a pediatric neurosurgeon at New York University (NYU). I also made a reservation at Boston Children's Hospital. I was so appreciative of Dr. Britton's quick response and referral.

Dr. Epstein was able to tamp down our fears with the statement I will remember for the rest of my life: "I can get this, and it won't grow back."

I canceled my trip to Boston. Ryan had a subarachnoid cyst (a sac filled with spinal fluid that is located between the brain or spinal cord) and not cancer. I am forever grateful that he was the only baby in the neonatal ICU that did not have cancer.

The surgery was successful, and my husband and I took our baby home within a week after his brain surgery. Ryan was in my arms still wearing the surgical dressing that covered his entire head. Our three-year-old, my favorite first-born son, was with the babysitter. When she opened the door, I expected a major hug, but much to my surprise, he started to scream in a very scared way and said, "Monster baby, Monster baby, that is not my brother Ryan. Take him outside and bring back my brother Ryan."

He ran to the kitchen, and I followed him and tried to hug him, but he was so scared. He sat down across from me, and I remember saying, "If I have to put the mon . . . your brother Ryan outside then he would be alone, and if I stayed with him, you would be alone. So, we all have to go outside, or we all stay inside because your mom loves you both so much."

I had the babysitter take Ryan and I hugged my favorite first-born until he was no longer scared.

Ryan went on to be a national class swimmer, talented in mathematics, getting an almost perfect score on the math section of the SAT, and a graduate from UC Berkeley. He is married to his beautiful wife Alicia and is now mother to my favorite first-born grandson, Miles Avery Emanuel. He is also co-founder and chief technology officer for Filmatic AI.

I could only imagine what would have happened if I was not a physician. Would my son have survived? In my situation, being a physician helped me to maneuver my way through the complicated health system during the most challenging time in my life. I was able to communicate with other physicians who were my friends and family, and most importantly Dr. Epstein, who was a caring and compassionate human being, an extremely knowledgeable, confident, and competent physician who was not afraid to say in no uncertain terms, "I can get this, and it won't grow back." He did not see my son as a Black baby, he saw my son as a baby who needed surgery to remove the subarachnoid cyst and he was committed to doing so.

I think Ryan's story also sheds light on health equity, and that conscious and unconscious bias is not embedded in all physicians, and health equity is attainable for all patients.

However, sadly, Black newborn babies in the United States are more likely to survive childbirth if they are cared for by Black doctors, but three times more likely than White babies to die when looked after by White doctors, a study has found. Researchers from George Mason University analyzed data capturing 1.8 million hospital births in Florida between 1992 and 2015 for the new study, which was published August 17, 2020, in the journal *Proceedings of the National Academy of Sciences of the United States of America*, also known as PNAS.[18]

When cared for by White physicians, Black newborns were about three times more likely to die in the hospital than White newborns, the researchers found. That disparity dropped significantly when the doctor was Black, although Black newborns nonetheless remained more likely than White newborns to die. The mortality rate of Black newborns in hospitals shrunk by between 39-58 percent when Black physicians took charge of the birth, according to the research, which laid bare how shocking racial disparities in human health can affect even the first hours of a person's life. By contrast, the mortality rate for White babies was largely unaffected by the doctor's race.

---

18 Greenwood, Brad N., Rachel R. Hardeman, Laura Huang, and Aaron Sojourner. "Physician—Patient Racial Concordance and Disparities in Birthing Mortality for Newborns." *Proceedings of the National Academy of Sciences* 117, no. 35 (2020): 21194—200. https://doi.org/10.1073/pnas.1913405117. Greenwood, Brad N., Rachel R. Hardeman, Laura Huang, and Aaron Sojourner. "Physician—Patient Racial Concordance and Disparities in Birthing Mortality for Newborns." *Proceedings of the National Academy of Sciences* 117, no. 35 (August 17, 2020): 21194—200. https://doi.org/10.1073/pnas.1913405117.

"Our study provides the first evidence that the Black-White newborn mortality gap is smaller when Black M.D.s provide care for Black newborns than when White M.D.s do, lending support to research examining the importance of racial concordance in addressing healthcare inequities," co-author Rachel Hardeman said on X (formerly Twitter). "Black babies have been dying at disproportionate rates since as long as we've collected data. The time is now to change this and to ensure that Black infants are afforded the opportunity to thrive."

I shared my story with Roger Shields, our twenty-three-year-old diagnosed with CHF, whom the team referred to as "Our Baby" with the hope that he would realize that his disease does not define who he is, and that the disease does not represent the totality of who he is as an individual human being. He had no family member that was a physician or employed in any area of healthcare.

The team who was committed to improving the healthcare of an individual showed the same level of empathy, caring, and competence to Roger in a nonjudgmental manner.

Roger's Story—Our Baby

Twenty-three-year-old Roger S was presented to the Kings Hospital ED in March 2012 with upper respiratory infection symptoms. Aside from being grossly overweight, Roger had no previous medical problems. He was treated by the emergency room staff and released that day. When he returned in April coughing up sputum, he was treated with antibiotics and again sent home. Then, in May, Roger again appeared in the ED, this time with shortness of breath and swollen legs, which was diagnosed as new-onset congestive heart failure. Looking at the X-rays from his emergency room visits after he was admitted to the hospital, they could see his heart enlarging.

That's when Roger was sent to my team on D4 South, where the cardiologist, looking at echocardiograms and other studies, was able to identify the underlying cause of Roger's heart failure as viral myocarditis—a viral infection of the heart muscle.

I will never forget Roger's parents crying that day.

"What has happened to my son?" were his father's words.

"I thought heart failure is for old people," his mother cried.

And young Roger's words, "What can I do to live?"

It was at that point that Roger became our team's "Baby."

We never thought we would have a twenty-three-year-old congestive heart failure patient. It was an emotional experience for all of us. It soon became apparent that the typical discharge with follow-up appointments and medication education was not going to be enough. Roger needed handholding, management of his fears, and constant communication with both his doctors and his parents.

Under the cardiologist's assurance that if Roger lost one hundred pounds, his ejection fraction would come back up, indicating that his heart was once again pumping a healthy amount of blood.

Roger was an assistant chef and with a dietician and homecare visits, made changes to his diet and managed his portions in such a way that by November he had lost one hundred pounds. Then he called us in December to say that he was moving to New Mexico. That's when Esther, the social worker on the team, came up with a barrage of questions: "Who's going to be your doctor? Who's going to manage your medications? What about your insurance coverage?" We had gotten him Managed Medicaid to cover his cost of treatment at Kings.

And finally, "You are not going!" Esther said.

His response, "I am an adult!"

Esther, "Oh, really. Is that a fact? And who gave you that diagnosis? Your diagnosis is heart failure!"

Roger wound up going to New Mexico to start a food truck on the college campus where his girlfriend was a student and we continued to communicate with him. But the drama was not over.

Five years later, after returning to New York, Roger called me one day to say that he wasn't feeling well. By then, I was no longer at New York Health + Hospitals. I told him to go right to the emergency room, and once again he was admitted to D4 South. When I called the next day, I was informed that he had been transferred to Bellevue Hospital in case he needed surgery. His diagnosis: intracerebral bleeding. And his INR was elevated, which measures blood thinning. I suspect they had probably put him on blood thinners because they suspected a thromboembolism, or a blood clot in the lungs. Hence the brain hemorrhage. And he was in heart failure.

When I arrived at Bellevue, I found Roger intubated and unconscious. He had total system failure. His liver failed, his kidney failed, his brain failed, his heart failed, and he had bilateral pneumonia.

The low point, as I saw it, came when one of the Bellevue interns assumed he must be a drug abuser.

"What makes you think he's using drugs?" I asked.

"Because he has blood in his finger," she replied.

"What do you mean?" I asked. "His INR is elevated, so his blood is thin, and he is bleeding. So, if he has something coming out of his finger, why would you assume he's a drug addict? How many drug addicts do you see who shoot up in their thumb?"

It was because he was Black. That's why I thought she was thinking that. This conversation with the intern was not representative of the care Roger received from the Bellevue team. They were very caring, compassionate, empathetic, and provided the best care imaginable. From the beginning, even though he was in total body failure, they had hopes that he would recover and were committed to helping him recover, which he did. To quote a member of the team, "He is an amazing individual!"

To make a long story short, on a regular basis, I would take the train down to Bellevue to visit Roger, and two weeks later, he woke up.

"Roger," I said, "do you know who I am?"

"Dr. B!" he called to me.

And there I was talking to him. "You've been out of it," I said. "You've been in a coma. We couldn't talk to you."

And he said, "Dr. B, I couldn't communicate with anyone, but I was communicating with myself."

"What do you mean?" I asked.

"I kept seeing my father, and he was in the military," he said. "I kept seeing my father and talking to my father." I was stunned at his statement, as I never heard before from Roger, that when in coma, self-communication was a part of the mindset.

His return was a miracle, his doctor said, as was his recovery after rehab, where he overcame his hemiparesis, or paralysis of his right side, and was restored to full function.

Twenty-three-year-old Roger Shields. When I think of him, I think of the miracles that can be achieved through exceptional medical care coupled with human value, empathy, and non-judgmental patient engagement.

SECTION II

CHAPTER 7

Nine Simple Solutions for Addressing Health Disparities and Achieving Health Equity

Health equity can be achievable if we can begin by recognizing, respecting, and valuing all patients as human beings. Health equity ensures everyone has a fair and just opportunity to be as healthy as possible. It means everyone having the opportunity to attain their full or optimal physical and mental health potential with the right conditions, and resources without any bias or stereotypes or barriers. There is huge evidence that health disparities have continued to adversely impact groups of people who experience greater obstacles to their health, based on their racial or ethnic group, socioeconomic status or other social or physical qualities. Health disparities are unfair differences that are intricately linked with social, economic and/or environmental disadvantage.[19]

In this chapter, I offer simple solutions and strategies for moving the dial toward health equity and assuring progress toward equitable health outcomes for all patients.

---

[19] Braveman P. What are health disparities and health equity? We need to be clear. Public Health Rep. 2014 Jan-Feb;129 Suppl 2(Suppl 2):5-8. doi: 10.1177/00333549141291S203. PMID: 24385658; PMCID: PMC3863701. Braveman, Paula. "What Are Health Disparities and Health Equity? We Need to Be Clear." *Public Health Reports* 129, no. 1_suppl2 (January 2014): 5—8. https://doi.org/10.1177/00333549141291s203.

The nine solutions highlighted in the table below center around patient engagement and prioritizing the human experience and value as individuals.

Solution Strategy

1. Patient Engagement and Cultural Sensitivity Training for clinical, executive leadership team and administrative staff.
2. Heighten human value for all patients through the concept of The Common Thread: The Human Experience
3. Never use noncompliant or nonadherent without asking the "Why" question
4. Eliminate the term "drug seeker" when describing individuals with Sickle Cell disease
5. Provide a comprehensive Social History
6. Application of The Spot Check Methodology
7. Application of the CHANGE Mnemonic
8. Application of similar surveys to patient and clinical teams
9. Self-reflection practice on being a patient in a hospital

1. Patient Engagement and Cultural Sensitivity Training Program

Building engagement with patients is a process that requires an awareness and knowledge of individual human value. It also includes knowledge of how culture and belief systems shape health and behaviors, as well as skills to identify strategies to incorporate cultural insights into practice. Culture in this instance refers to the integrated patterns of human behavior such as language, customs, beliefs, thoughts, actions, values, experiences, and institutions that are practiced by a group of people. As such, culture can influence a patient's view of their illness and what caused it, their attitudes toward doctors or other healthcare providers, and when to decide to seek healthcare.

Cultural sensitivity is defined as the ability of providers and hospitals to effectively deliver healthcare services that meet the social, cultural, and linguistic needs of patients. A culturally competent healthcare system can help improve health outcomes and quality of care and can contribute to the elimination of racial and ethnic health disparities. The cultural sensitivity training program recognizes that we as healthcare professionals need to educate ourselves and recognize that our beliefs and attitudes, conscious or unconscious, can have a positive or negative impact on patient care and compliance, the patient experience, self-management, and health outcomes.

The Power of Patient Engagement and Cultural Sensitivity: An Inter-cultural Communication Approach

There are many cultures at work within each healthcare encounter or visit in which patient engagement occurs. This includes the patient's culture, the healthcare provider's culture, the culture of the healthcare institution and the culture of the practice of medicine in itself. This is important to understand since each personal culture embraces what is regarded as meaningful—their values, experiences, preferences or assumptions about perception or reality.

In addition to understanding and awareness of patient cultures, there is a need for purposeful cultural sensitivity training of foreign medical graduates, American-born and trained physicians to foreign-born and American-born patients.

Current statistics show that one in five physicians are born and educated abroad.[20] In other US states that rely heavily on foreign doctors, the percentage ranges from 32 percent (California, Maryland, and District of Columbia) or 33 percent (New York), to 37 percent (New Jersey).[21] If that foreign-born physician is accepted in a health

---
20 AAMC Professional Physician Data (AAMC) Masterfile May 23, 2023
21 Immigrant Healthcare Workers in the United States. Migration Policy Institute April 7, 2023, 20

system that's toxic to Black patients, it's likely that they will adopt the negativity. We need to understand the role of race/gender in American culture and race and/or gender in foreign cultures. The English-speaking Black population is currently left out of the cultural competence requirement and conversation.

The inter-cultural communication and cultural sensitivity approach will consist of:

- **Foreign medical graduates to American-born patients:** the need to understand the positives and negatives of the American healthcare system and the health disparity that Black patients endure. If the culture of the health system is toxic, they will join in and be a part of the problem.
- **American-born physicians to foreign-born patients:** and the need to recognize the need for language support, cultural sensitivity, and delivery of excellent healthcare irrespective of immigration status. American physicians need to understand cultural norms that are different from American norms. American physicians need to understand the role of the caregiver. The caregiver may not be the decision-maker in other cultures. They also need to understand the role of doctors in other societies. For example, the "I say it, you do it" philosophy.
- **American-born physicians to American-born patients:** the need to recognize the cultural and linguistic diversity among patients, including diverse lived experiences, which can translate to beliefs about the healthcare system, whether medically sound or not.

Given that each patient is a unique individual, these cross-cultural bi-directional approaches need targeted strategies to uncover the cultural preferences and frames of reference.

Cultural sensitivity training must be applied across the board to be inclusive of all patient populations, including English-speaking, limited English proficiency, and non-English-speaking populations. Currently, the English-speaking population is left out of the conversation.

A comprehensive training program must be a part of the Human Resources employee training processes. The training needs to be implemented for all clinical departments including nurses, social workers, care/case managers, patient experience officers, and administrators. The training exercise should include how assumptions, biases, and the provider's frame of reference (or stereotypes) result in barriers to optimal patient engagement and health outcomes. An example of a strategy includes making the wrong assumptions and perceptions about patients or patient groups, which are often different from the reality of the population served and/or the individual human being.

2. The Common Thread: The Human Experience

When an individual receives a diagnosis accurately, the disease or condition is non-negotiable and cannot be given back and may remain with the individual for life. Irrespective of race, gender, age, socioeconomic status, or country of origin, it cannot be given back and may remain with the individual for life. It applies to all human beings whether they are a millionaire or homeless. The millionaire can't say, "I will give you a million dollars to take the cancer back; oh, that's not enough? I will give you five million."

The option of having choices is eliminated totally, unlike in all other aspects of life where we may have choices. If you don't like the school your children attend, if you don't like your job, or if you don't like your family, you have choices. These are examples of choices we have in life. Therefore, having empathy toward a patient with a disease diagnosis, rather than a judgmental attitude, is the morally appropriate approach to providing clinical care.

If a health system improves the health of the most vulnerable population, then it can improve the health of all populations. Amid diversity, the common thread is "The Human Experience" of dealing with a non-negotiable disease. Recognition that the disease is not the "sum total" of the individual is essential. The word "patient" does not fully understand and address the complexity of the individual human being. Patient value and quality of life is a "no-brainer."

Physician's Approach to the Common Thread

- American and foreign-born physicians can develop a shared understanding.
- Patients, irrespective of birthplace, language, religious beliefs, and appearance, voluntarily came to our institutions.
- They may have received a diagnosis that they did not want and one which is non-negotiable.
- The possibility of the disease being a lifelong burden requires major lifestyle changes.
- Appreciation that there may be a need to understand where the patient is in acceptance of the disease.

Faced with a diagnosis or disease condition, what do the *diverse* patients have in common?
Below are some key points to keep in mind.

- They don't have choices about their diseases. Once diagnosed accurately, the disease is NON- NEGOTIABLE.
- They can't give the disease back—the concept is that once accurately diagnosed, one can't say "I don't want it" and give it back.
- In the case of chronic conditions, the disease and its symptoms may remain with patients for life.

- Patients may be forced to change their lifestyle and/or job as a result of the disease.
- They may experience temporary or permanent loss of control over their life.
- At any point in our lives, we as health professionals may become patients

A major accomplishment toward achieving health equity will be to have an enriched cultural sensitivity and patient engagement experience that would occur regardless of the patient's socioeconomic status, race, ethnicity, health status or disease condition, at the point of care. Ideally, when an inpatient admission occurs, it should be because there is a serious life-threatening problem. Far too often, our inability to better communicate, listen to, and engage with the patient as an individual human being, and in a culturally sensitive manner, results in suboptimal care, medical treatment, unnecessary hospitalization, and adverse health outcomes.

3. Never use Noncompliant/Nonadherent without Asking the "Why" Question

Commit to never using the word noncompliant without asking "Why?" If the clinical team does not know the reasons an individual did not take their medication or did not follow recommendations and/or directions, they need to inquire why before labeling the patient noncompliant. It often happens that the same medication regimen that the patient was not able to follow, is often prescribed again. The question is: Can clinical care be effective and the individual's health outcome be in the positive direction without the "Why" question to address any treatment compliance concerns? The "Why" question is crucial, as it could potentially eliminate conscious or unconscious bias as well as wrongful staff perceptions. Improved communication and engagement help to promote and create an environment of empathy, as opposed to negative judgmental attitudes from the clinical teams.

Proposed Questions for Patients to Discuss with their Doctor.

If you did not follow directions and your doctor did not ask "WHY"

- Do you want to know why I didn't follow directions?
- Did you write noncompliant or nonadherent in my medical record?
- Please delete noncompliant, nonadherent in my medical record if you don't include "Why."
- Do you realize that negative language in my medical record can impact my health outcome?

4. Eliminate the Term "drug seekers" when Describing Individuals with Sickle Cell Disease.

Patients with Sickle Cell disease suffer two types of pain. The unimaginable physical pain that results from the vaso-occlusive crisis, which occurs when sickled red blood cells block blood flow to the point that tissues become deprived of oxygen, is the most prevalent. The second type of pain is the mental and emotional pain that occurs when patients are in such physically painful crises and are being referred to, inappropriately, as "drug seekers." This emotional and mental pain is unwarranted and unnecessary. It is the result of either conscious or unconscious bias due to a lack of compassion and empathy on the part of healthcare providers toward this population. All care providers should eliminate the term "drug seeker," as it is not supported by medical literature.

I would recommend the following conversation for patients with SCD to have with their clinical team, when they are in the emergency room and not getting the timely and needed care that they are entitled to and deserve.

Individuals with Sickle Cell Disease: Conversation with Physicians and the Clinical Team

If you are unable to speak because of the unimaginable pain, have a family member or your advocate ask these questions or have the conversations on your behalf.

1. I am a human being who happens to be African American. I have a life-threatening disorder, SCD, and I am in severe pain and I need to be valued and treated Now!

2. Like you, I have dreams and aspirations, so please do not cut my life short because you don't value me.

3. If you do not receive an acceptable response, ask to speak with the Emergency Medical Director.

4. Make sure you have a referral to a hematologist and primary care physician upon discharge from the emergency department.

5. If you are hospitalized, ask to speak to a behavioral health specialist to be able to discuss your feelings, fears, anxiety, depression, family circumstances and anything that's important to you.

6. Make sure you have a follow-up appointment on discharge from the hospital.

7. You don't have to feel uncomfortable requesting a mental health counselor. It should be a vital part of your treatment for SCD.

8. Mental health counseling is recognized as a need in other life-threatening diseases such as cystic fibrosis, so why not SCD?

Important Statement to Keep in Your Phone

Keep the quote below in your phone. If needed, show it to the clinical team and ask them not to do unpleasant things to worsen your medical condition.

In the words of Dr. William T. Zempsky, a leading pain researcher, "Difficult patients are not just born, they are in part created by their passage through the medical system. Not only has this system failed to cure them, but it may also have done unpleasant things to make matters worse."

1 Zempsky, William T. "Treatment of Sickle Cell Pain." JAMA 302, no. 22 (2009):2479. https://doi.org/10.1001/jama.2009.1811.

5. Provide a Comprehensive Social History

During medical school training, we are taught to include as much background sociodemographic information about the patient as possible. This means including information about the patient's occupation or job status, marital status, living arrangements, education level, and religion, as well as the use of drugs, alcohol, or tobacco. We were discouraged by how limited the social history was, as it only stated *non-drinker, non-smoker,* or *no toxic substances.* This was unacceptable. Sadly, this is the case in a significant number of patients' social history in today's medical records. It is important for the social history of individual patients to include as much background demographic information, including their values, how they describe themselves, and their accomplishments. Familiarity with a patient's social history is one of the first steps in getting to know the individual as a person. The notion that an African American elderly individual who has been in church since birth is now being described as a 'non-drinker,' 'non-smoker,' or an individual with "no history of toxic substance use" is unconscionable.

6. Application of The Spot Check Methodology

The Spot (Speak, Pacify, Outline, Take) check methodology is a framework to help to better understand and manage the patient with a new diagnosis of a disease or condition. The method includes key questions that clinical teams, patients, and families can use to better understand their fears about receiving a new diagnosis, identify what is important to them, where they are in terms of acceptance of the diagnosis, and help alleviate any concerns.

Purpose of the questions for clinical teams:
a) **Speak** to patients and families
b) **Pacify** fears
c) **Outline** what is important to the individual
d) **Take** into consideration where the individual is in the acceptance of the disease

Questions posed to each patient should include:
1. Who am I as an individual?
2. What are my fears?
3. What is important to me?
4. Where am I in the acceptance of my diagnosis?

Purpose of the questions for patients: When an individual is given an unexpected diagnosis of a disease or condition that could be life-threatening, oftentimes there is no preparation for coping. This is what I refer to as the non-negotiable disease. There is confusion and fear, amidst not having a coping mechanism. The questions for the patients are designed to help staff better understand the patients as individuals, their fears, what's important to them, and the phase of acceptance of the diagnosis. Equally important is to share the information gathered with their healthcare providers. They need to know who the patient is, as an individual, and that being a patient is only a part of the individual they are.

Spot Check Methodology

General Outline	Questions posed to each patient should include: 1. Who am I as an individual? 2. What are my fears? 3. What's important to me? 4. Where am I in the acceptance of my diagnosis?
Speak to patient/family to understand the individual	Who is the individual (Married/Single/Separated/ Divorced; Mother/Wife/Grandmother/Widow; Father/Husband/Grandfather/Widower; Educational level/Employment; Place of Birth; English-speaking, non-English speaking, limited English proficiency, bi/multilingual; belief system)?
Pacify fear factors if possible	What are the fear factors that keep the individual up at night? (e.g., Am I going to die? Will the treatment make me feel worse? Can I have a normal life? Is this my fault? Did God do this to me?).
Outline what is important to the individual	Family, Work, Character, Religion/Culture/Ethnicity, Finance, Health, Fun and Recreation, Privacy, Dignity and Respect, Choices.
Take into consideration the time it takes an individual to accept the disease	Where is the individual in the acceptance of the disease? Are they in denial and how do we as health professionals put forth a plan to help the individual in the acceptance of the disease?

The importance of obtaining patient responses to the questions is multifaceted. It includes getting an understanding of the fear factors—and possibly lack of acceptance—of the disease that can potentially drive "noncompliance," knowing who the individual patient is, and what is important to them. This level of communication and engagement is a game changer. In addition to driving better engagement, it can increase trust and collaboration between patients and families, improve health outcomes, and drive better compliance.

7. Application of the CHANGE Mnemonic

The CHANGE mnemonic is a way of addressing biases and false assumptions about patients and engaging them in a culturally sensitive manner.

CHANGE mnemonic

C	Change negative perceptions and wrong assumptions about patient by seeking to understand the reality
H	How can I help?
A	Acknowledge the atrocities that were endured by Black patients and their families, and in particular the elderly Black patient.
N	Never Use Noncompliant without asking why.
G	Give the patient the benefit of the doubt.
E	Empathetic Care should be at the center of patient engagement.

Acknowledging the history of atrocities that the elderly Black population suffered is unique only to this population and should be recognized and understood. Patient Voice: My parents were a step away from slavery and my grandparents were slaves.

For example, in discussion with a patient about taking medications or about their diagnosis, if you get the response, **"I don't trust you doctors,"** try the following:

> **Response**: "Tell me about your healthcare experience." If it's horrible then you may want to apologize, show empathy, and add, "I don't know if I could have dealt with it. But here is why you have x condition and let me tell you why."
>
> **Rationale**: You want to get the patient out of the past and into the here and now.

8. Application of Similar Surveys to Patients and Clinical Teams

When applying the HCAHPS questionnaire patients are asked: What do patients think about the care they received? Would they recommend the hospital?

Equally important would be to develop a survey to determine what the staff thinks about the population they serve. If staff opinion is negative, it can potentially affect HCAP Scores. If the staff survey results are based on perception versus reality of the population served, it could potentially impact the HCAHP scores either positively or negatively.

Examples of staff survey questions to address perception or reality.

- What percentage of patients are insured?
- What percentage of patients go to shelters?
- What percentage of patients are believed to be noncompliant?
- What percentage of patients understand the instructions given?
- What percentage of patients are deemed to be illiterate?
- What percentage of patients do you think follow directions?

Self-reflection Practice on Being a Patient in a Hospital Bed

It would be important for medical students and interns to reflect on what it's like to be in a hospital bed before starting clinical rotation at a hospital. How would it feel to have multiple clinical staff including physicians, social workers, and nurses talking to you throughout the day and night?

- Do I understand the conversation as it's being spoken in medical terms?
- When my surgery canceled and I have been NPO for ten to twelve hours, what happens to all the medications I am being given? Are there any side effects?

- The patient coded in the bed next to me.
- What is the impact of my age on how valuable I am being viewed? On my diagnosis? Is my race and/or ethnicity viewed as positive or negative?
- How do I communicate in my primary language? What if the clinical team feels negatively toward me?
- What if I fall?
- What if I develop an infection in the hospital?
- If I am African American, how would I feel as I am not a part of the cultural sensitivity conversation?

Purpose of role-playing exercise

- For medical or health professional students to understand what it's like for individuals to obtain needed healthcare starting in the emergency room, and the trials and tribulations to get to the inpatient unit.
- Recognize the mental and emotional understanding of being a patient inclusive of patient fears.
- The importance of knowing the individual.
- Become more empathetic and less judgmental of patients irrespective of race, gender, religion, or ethnicity.
- Heighten human value.
- Provide more empathetic and compassionate care.
- Address unconscious and conscious bias

The self-reflection would cause participants to think about how traumatic and difficult it is to be a hospitalized patient. This self-reflection can help you to better communicate with patients, and as a result improve engagement, be less judgmental of patients, and promote better health outcomes. The application of the nine solutions to obtain health equity is a guide to clinicians and patients. Once it's operationalized, it will have a major positive effect on eliminating health disparity that is perpetuated by conscious or unconscious biases. This could also result in increased empathy and an increase in acknowledging or prioritizing human value.

What Have We Learned?

- Behavioral change starts with healthcare professionals and executives.
- Professionals and patients share the same human concerns and emotions.
- Religion, ethnicity, race, gender, and culture trumps illness.
- Historical trauma can influence patient behavior.
- Terms such as "Frequent Flyers" and "Noncompliant/Adherent" used over time in a healthcare setting toward patients can create a culture of callous disregard.
- A culture of callous disregard can negatively impact patient health and safety, and thus affect patient compliance.
- That we all can become patients at any given point in time.

Staff instructions from a patient

Example: A Caribbean patient with hypertension who believes herbal remedies are best to treat his medical condition stated, "For me to change from the 'Bush Tea' (traditional cultural home remedy), you have to tell me the severity of why you want to add one or two medications. If you want me to take three or four medications you have to personalize it, man!

Patient centered care—who knew?!

During a patient's two-week follow-up appointment with his cardiologist, he informed me, his doctor, that he was having trouble with one of his medications.

"Which one?" I asked.

"The patch. The nurse told me to put on a new one every six hours and now I'm running out of places to put it!"

I had him quickly undress and discovered what I had hoped I wouldn't see. Yes, the man had over fifty patches on his body! Now, the instructions included removal of the old patch before applying a new one.

If any healthcare institution and/or medical school would be interested in implementing the pilot program, please contact me at mbeverleymd@gmail.com.

The application of the nine solutions to obtain health equity is a guide to clinicians and patients. Once it's operationalized in health systems, it will have a major positive effect on eliminating health disparity based on biases, conscious or unconscious, and as a result increase human value of all populations. That could be the second common thread.

CHAPTER 8

Improving the Patient Engagement and Cultural Competence Experience Training: A Road Map

Background

Healthcare delivery systems are evolving with a focus on changing patients' behavior to improve access, utilization, and health outcomes. Less attention has been paid to the needed behavioral changes of healthcare professionals, as our attitudes impact patient care.

This training program is comprehensive in its approach and is designed to improve the patient's care and experience in a culturally competent manner.

Purpose

We as healthcare professionals and executive administrators need to recognize that our beliefs and attitudes, conscious or unconscious, can have a positive or negative impact on: (i) Patient care and compliance, (ii) The patient experience, (iii) Self-management, and (iv) Health outcomes.

A patient engagement and cultural competence experience training is essential for all healthcare providers to:

- Increase empathy.
- Respect and understand the individual's cultural beliefs regarding their health.
- Prevent judgmental behavior directed at patients.
- Prevent disparate care.
- Maintain patient dignity.
- Improve the health outcomes for the elderly Black population.

Self-Evaluation

Healthcare administrators and providers need to better understand the ways in which our own biases, values and beliefs can impact our perceptions and decisions, and influence on patient care.

How do we as healthcare administrators and professionals want to be viewed?	Identifying Our Cultural Beliefs and Attitudes	Are Patients Really Different From Us as Individuals?
	What do we as individuals value?	Patients as individuals also value:
• Professional • Knowledgeable • Honest • Caring • Open Minded • Nonjudgmental • Problem Solver • Culturally Competent	• Self • Family • Work • Integrity • Religion/Culture/Ethnicity • Finance • Health • Fun and Recreation • Privacy • Dignity and Respect • Choices	• Family • Work • Character • Religion/Culture/Ethnicity • Finance • Health • Fun and Recreation • Privacy • Dignity and Respect • Choices

Language of Negativity: Does it reflect high patient value?

It's important to recognize that the language of negativity is a major contributor to health disparity and as a result the lack of human value.

- **Noncompliant**—The term noncompliant is generally used to refer to a patient who intentionally refuses to take a prescribed treatment or care plan and does not follow the recommendations that have been given by the doctor or care team. Using this label for patients, without asking "Why"—it's the catalyst to being dismissive to patients, particularly Black patients. Negative language written in the medical record will create a culture where the patient has to navigate himself or herself through an overly complicated health system and as a result increase negative language to "frequent flyer."

- **Frequent Flyer**—The term "frequent flyer" is used to label patients who become repeat visitors to the emergency department or hospital because of a chronic illness, or most often regarded as though they are seeking medical attention. This is a pejorative branding since the patients are often assumed to be problem patients. In some settings, they are seen to be malingerers, or drug seekers. This label results in a total lack of interest or empathy toward the individual. I am of the opinion as I stated that noncompliant without the "Why" may create Frequent Flyers.

- **High Utilizer**—This term refers to patients that hospitals regard as imposing a disproportionately high burden and prohibitive cost to their services because of their frequent ED and hospital resource use. Deserving of punishment.

- **Drug Seekers**—As the name implies, this term refers to patients who are seen as "gaming the system" in order to satisfy their drug addiction needs. This is an unfair characterization and perpetuates the lack of empathy for patients. Most often Sickle Cell patients are labeled drug seekers—a wrong categorization of Sickle Cell patients, which is not supported in the medical literature.

All of these create a culture of callous disregard and can possibly contribute to poor health outcomes.

Counter-Productive Thought Process

Physicians and Nurses are trained to ask questions. Not asking reasons "Why," is counter to medical training and the analytical thought processes.

Language of Negativity—Its Impact

The impact of negative language may:
- Cause potential adverse health outcomes.
- Cause repetitive ED visits.
- Cause increased readmissions.
- Increase healthcare costs.
- Limit willingness to educate patients.
- Increase the health burden for patients.
- Required consents may not be given.
- Detached from the patient engagement process.
- If the patient is not valued:
- We may not be as effective in explaining medical issues and medication as well as we should.
- We may not engage the family.
- We may (un)intentionally influence other staff behavior.

- We may unintentionally substitute "Do no harm" for harm.
- "Frequent Flyers" implies that the patients are no longer valued as human beings.

Some important activities:
- Determine the percentage of patients in your facility that you label noncompliant without asking "Why."
- Address the skewed language in the patient's social history—non-drinker, non-smoker, no toxic substance—that unfairly defines the individual. If a patient describes themselves as a church-going African American female retired postal worker and teacher, that's how she should be described. It is unconscionable to reduce a patient's social history to whether they drink, smoke, or use substances.

The Importance of Social History

A social history should provide a comprehensive picture **about the** individual **patient, including a subjective description of how they want to be** perceived.

CHECKLIST
- Is it comprehensive in describing the individual?
- Is the individual only being defined as: Non-drinker, non-smoker, or no toxic substance?
- The combination of noncompliant/nonadherent without asking "Why." coupled with "No toxic substance" is now defining a human being.

Limiting social history devalues the important aspects of the individual patient. However, we are taught in medical school what should be included in social history.

If one's perception of the individual is the same as the reality, then there is an opportunity to make necessary changes. But if one's perception is different from the reality, we run the risk of increasing disparity in care and health outcomes.

Eradicating Misperceptions and Fallacies

In healthcare it's not unusual for the African American population, irrespective of socioeconomic status, to **be stereotyped and given wrong assumptions or** perceptions **about who they really are.**

An Example of a Perception Versus Reality

The COVID Pandemic has shed a bright light on the long-standing numerous health inequities experienced by Black Americans across the US The Black population has the highest COVID-19 death rate.

PERCEPTION:

The prevailing thought is that it's a result of poverty, lack of access to care, social determinants of health, and comorbidities.

REALITY:

For example, Prince George County in Maryland, one of the wealthiest Black upper-class communities in the nation, has some of the highest COVID-19 mortality.

Brooklyn, NY, with a large Black population, thirteen hospitals including three public and one state hospital and extensive public transportation has the highest COVID-associated deaths in New York City.

Public transportation employees who died were predominantly Black union workers with an average salary of approximately $50,000, with pensions and health coverage.

Perception: Patients with Sickle Cell Disease have a higher degree of drug addiction than the general population

Fact: Opioid addiction for patients with Sickle Cell disease ranges from 0.5 to 8 percent vs. 3 to 16 percent in patients with other chronic pain syndromes. Behaviors often described for patients with Sickle Cell disease, such as requesting a specific dose of opioid or requesting that the opioid be administered intravenously, may be normative in patients who have experienced a history of undertreatment of pain. These are less indicative of abuse, compared with behaviors for opioid requests in illicit drug use or opioid abuse for addictive symptoms other than pain.

Electronic Health Records: Can Negative Information Go Viral?

An electronic health record (EHR) that has complete, accurate, reliable, and comprehensive information has the potential to help providers diagnose a patient's problem sooner, implement the right supportive interventions or treatment and improve patient outcomes. It also can prevent adverse events or medical errors if there are risk management or alerts in place. The information that is currently gathered by a primary physician or clinical care team and recorded in the EHR is useful in informing other providers accordingly. As such, information about a patient is critical. Erroneous information about a patient is a quality and safety issue. Biased or stereotypical information can also cause harm. Currently, multiple health systems share their electronic health records within their networks.

Some questions to reflect on include: Is there a positive or negative association with patient engagement and experience that is being transcribed in the EHR? Will it improve health outcomes when EHRs are fed negative terminology in describing patients? Will the receiving subspecialist, nurse, social workers, and receptionist want to engage patients that are described as frequent flyers, noncompliant/

adherents, and drug seekers? How soon will that individual get a needed appointment with a sub-specialist with such negative terminology about them?

Internet Accessibility

Is the internet currently a source of health and disease information that supersedes physician expertise? Is the internet the driver of healthcare, as opposed to healthcare professionals? Are patients and families following directions from their providers or the internet?

Are our sons and daughters in high school and college in the chat rooms making decisions about their health? What percentage of healthcare is being accessed through the internet? Do we know?

Organizational Cultural Competency

Organizational cultural competency is defined as the ability of providers and organizations to effectively deliver healthcare services that meet social, cultural, and linguistic needs of patients. A culturally competent healthcare system can help improve health outcomes and quality of care and can contribute to the elimination of racial and ethnic health disparities.

Need for a New Approach and Communication with Patients

ASK THE QUESTION:

What is the patient not saying that the healthcare providers are not hearing?
- I am embarrassed to talk about my living arrangements.
- I have not accepted the disease.
- I don't understand what you are saying.
- I can't afford the medications.
- I am scared to death about my condition.

- I am worried about the impact on my job and finances.
- I don't trust the medicines and I'm going to try home remedies

What is the physician, nurse or care manager not saying that the patient is hearing?
- I am not smart enough to understand my disease.
- I am in the low literacy group; therefore, I have low intelligence capability.
- You don't think that I am going to follow your instructions.
- "You people" don't usually follow instructions.
- You don't see the need to value and understand my cultural beliefs.
- You don't see me as valuable as you

Result: I may not receive the empathy, time, and resources to help me improve my health.
- Maintain patient dignity while asking probing questions about medical history, personal habits, and behaviors.
- Body Language—universal communication tool in a diverse patient population.
- Continuous improvement in cultural competence.
- Be conscious of the time required for patients to come to terms with and accept his or her disease.
- Understand that patients have no choice but to accept their diagnosis and may need help coping with the disease and its impact on their lives and the lives of their loved ones

For example, if a patient is planning a vacation with family and their yearly mammogram is now abnormal, that individual may not even know who they are at this unexpected scary, and difficult point in their life.

Fear Factors—The Universal Thread

ASK THE QUESTION:

Patient Fear Factor
- Am I going to die?
- Will the treatment make me feel worse?
- Will I get better?
- Can I have a normal life?
- Is it my fault?
- Did God do this to me?

Family Fear Factor
- I don't have the resources to do this alone.
- I don't know if I can give the medications to a family member. What if I make a mistake? I could not live with myself if I made the medical condition of my family member worse.
- Can I afford not returning to work to care for a family member?
- What do I do if something goes wrong? Who can I call?

Patient Comments: Fear Factor
- Medication side effects may elicit more fear and discomfort than the disease itself.
- You are on your own after leaving the doctor's office.
- If the information about the side effects of the medication was not clearly communicated during the doctor visit, patients may not take their medication once the pharmacist explains the side effects.
- Patients may now be considered "noncompliant."
- Patients may be perceived as not caring about their own health

Understand that patients have no choice but to accept their diagnosis and they may need help coping with the disease and its impact on their lives and the lives of their loved ones

Question:
"Can you value my culture if you don't value me as an individual?"

Low Patient Value Can Possibly
- Turn competent professionals into incompetent professionals.
- Create a culture of callous disregard.
- Impact a patient's image of the institution.
- Compromise patient safety.
- Cause preventable adverse events

If the patient is not valued, then:
- We may be detached from the patient engagement process.
- We may not obtain the required consents.
- We may not be as effective in explaining medical issues and medication as well as we are capable of and should do.
- We may not engage the family.
- We may (un)intentionally influence other staff behavior.
- We may (un)intentionally substitute "Do no harm" for harm

Patient-Centered Care

Patient-centered care recognizes and treats patients not only from a clinical perspective but also from an emotional, mental, spiritual, social, and financial perspective.

Can we really label our practices "A Patient-Centered Medical Home" if:

- We continue to use negative language to describe individuals who are obtaining their medical care at our institutions.
- We don't apply the rules of cultural competence in delivering care to this community.

Patient-centered care starts with:
- Give the patient the benefit of the doubt.
- Be nonjudgmental.
- Have empathy.
- Eliminate use of negative labels such as high utilizers, drug seekers, frequent flyers, and noncompliant without knowing or asking "Why."
- Recognize that the average healthcare professional is healthier than the patient population and most have never been hospitalized.
- Those who were hospitalized tend to be women giving birth.
- Understand that we are trying to prevent the death of hospitalized patients.

Who are our patients? Not only are they English-speaking and American born, but they may also originate from different countries, speak different languages, and may have different religious beliefs. They may have different expectations regarding their healthcare needs and the role of healthcare providers and have different beliefs about the use of western medicine versus herbal and/or home remedies.

The Individual with a Disease versus the Disease Label

Care Management is about caring for individuals with one or more diseases, and as a result improving the health of the population. Care Management is not about broad-brushing a disease to a group of individuals.

EXAMPLE: DIABETES

When one says "diabetic," it may suggest "all diabetics are the same." The disease is the same, but the individuals with the disease are different.

FOR EXAMPLE

- A mother with two children managing her diabetes.
- A father who works twelve-hour shifts living with diabetes.
- A grandmother coping with her diagnosis of diabetes and who vehemently believes that she should leave the disease in "God's hands."
- For each of these three scenarios, Care Management would be vastly different and would require patient-centered and culturally sensitive engagement approaches.

CHAPTER 9

Six Scenarios for Health Systems and Healthcare Providers to Implement and Address

To move from health disparity to health equity, it is important for health systems to identify and address the six scenarios listed and the recommended solutions and strategies.

Scenario		Solution or Strategy
Scenario I Choices	Not to have patient choose between: - Health and family - Health and culture - Health and religious beliefs - Health and finance - Health and education	Patient choice is important and plays a significant role in deciding their own care and defining optimal care to meet their needs and overall wellbeing. The patient's wishes as well as the goals to provide quality, patient-centered care, should define the ethical obligations of the health provider to do no harm. Therefore, recognize that patients should not have to choose between their family, culture, religious beliefs, finance education and their health.
Scenario II	**Understanding the human response** and time required to accept a new diagnosis, we may need to engage in discussions about anger, denial, religious/cultural beliefs, and depression.	Providers may need to engage in discussions about anger, denial, religious/cultural beliefs, and depression and provide needed referrals for mental health counseling.

Scenario III	Understanding the role of historical racism and inequities of healthcare systems toward African Americans.	**Patient Concerns:** • They are not telling me what's wrong. • They don't treat me the same as Caucasians. • I don't really believe what they say. **Possible Response:** "You may not believe it, but you need to listen to me for your own health." **Preferred Response:** "Would you like to tell me about your or your family's experience with the healthcare system? Based on what you have just told me, I can empathize and understand why you feel that way. Here is why this experience is different."
Scenario IV	**Immigrant Perspective** • I should not question the doctor since he/she knows and understands health more than anyone. • All immigrants are not undocumented or uninsured. • Limited English proficiency and accents are not indicators of intelligence.	**For Low English Proficiency patients:** **Possible Responses:** •"Please repeat what I just said." •"Did you understand?" •"What part didn't you understand?" **Preferred Responses:** "I would like you to tell me whether you understood my instructions, as I may not have explained it as clearly as I should. Giving me feedback will also help me improve my communication with other patients."

Six Scenarios for Health Systems and Healthcare Providers to Implement and Address 127

Scenario V	**Senior Citizen Perception** • No longer of value. • Living on borrowed time. • Only limited communication is needed. **Mental Health** • The patient is a substance abuser—He or she is at fault, therefore he or she is of questionable human value. • They are "Frequent Flyers" abusing resources, falling on the floor, and don't know how to behave like a human being. • If they would only take their medications, they would not have "The Problem." • Seekers and abusers of certain prescription	The need to recognize the value of the elderly, particularly African Americans, when you consider the atrocities they have endured and continue to endure. Recognize when some patients need more help than others. Rather than negative labeling, the first response should be to discuss the need for mental health counseling in a humane and not judgmental manner. Recognize that we as individuals have different strengths and weaknesses at different times in our lives.
Scenario VI	**Challenge VI** **Staff Challenges** What kind of patient do you have difficulty in engaging in the care process? • Is it a non-verbal or non-communicative patient? • Is it an angry patient? • Is it _____? (Fill in the blank.) **What is your comfort level with patients who are:** • African Americans/African descent • Hispanic • Asian • Caucasian • American Indian • Mixed race • Male, female, transgender, LGBTQ	It's important to self-reflect and identify which type of patient applies to you. The need to recognize one's conscious or unconscious bias toward a particular individual or population served and the potential impact on health outcomes.

CONCLUSION

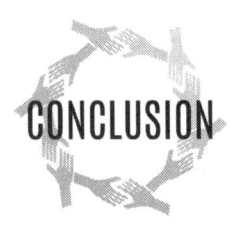

It's been an incredible journey in recognizing that there are simple boots-on-the-ground solutions to achieve health equity. It has been an eye-opening experience for me to realize that there is an opportunity to prevent escalation to the complex if we prevent and solve the simple problems in healthcare. Implementing health equity solutions required conventional and unconventional processes including instances such as stop-in-your-tracks moments, which were the voices of the patients in our hospital beds, in ambulatory care settings or in the emergency department.

As Deputy Executive Director, Care/Case Management at Kings County Hospital, it was humbling and a major learning experience hearing the voices of the elderly Black population with the recognition that the elderly Black population are in our hospital beds and not necessarily published in our history books. The realization that the English-speaking Black population, particularly the elderly Black population, were not included in the cultural sensitivity conversation was an unacceptable finding. I also realized that conversation on cultural competency needed to recognize and empathize with the atrocities the elderly Black population endured. The patients with Sickle Cell disease that signed up to be a part of our Sickle Cell Support Group were instrumental in changing the culture of the institution. Our results were amazing, and I am pleased that the Bridge Team is still operational at Elmhurst Hospital and the Sickle Cell Support Group is still operational at Queens Hospital.

The nine solutions are key game changers—moving the dial from health disparity to achieving health equity. The strategies are boots-on-the-ground solutions with the major focus on centering patients and their stories in discussions on health equity. Equally important is changing staff perception to the reality about the individual patient or population being served.

In terms of patient-centered care and cultural sensitivity training, the intent is to recognize that a culturally competent healthcare system can help improve health outcomes and quality of care and can contribute to the elimination of racial and ethnic health disparities. Cultural sensitivity training must be applied to: English-speaking, limited-English proficiency, and non-English-speaking populations. Currently, the English-speaking Black population is left out of the culturally competent training and conversation.

The human connection and valuing the human being are the first steps toward achieving health equity. If a human being is not valued, then that individual's healthcare is severely compromised and as a result a poor health outcome is inevitable.

It is crucial for patients to ask the "Why" question because more often than not, if the physician does not ask "Why," it then translates to negative language in the medical record, such as noncompliant/nonadherent, which can negatively impact one's health outcome.

Caregivers are an extension of their family members who require healthcare due to medical conditions. They are both inclusive and part of the process as well.

It is my hope that readers will find the content of this book and the nine solutions helpful for their health equity journey with patients. The time for achieving health equity is now, and we need to implement solutions that are simple and innovative.

SECTION III

RESOURCES

Health Disparities in the United States–Statistics

Disease Category	Outcome
Cardiovascular Disease	Death rates for African Americans remained 20 percent higher for heart disease and 40 percent higher for Cerebrovascular Accidents (CVA). Mensah, George A. "Cardiovascular Diseases in African Americans: Fostering Community Partnerships to Stem the Tide." American Journal of Kidney Diseases 72, no. 5 (2018). https://doi.org/10.1053/j.ajkd.2018.06.026. GA;, Mensah. "Cardiovascular Diseases in African Americans: Fostering Community Partnerships to Stem the Tide." American journal of kidney diseases : the official journal of the National Kidney Foundation. Accessed February 5, 2024. https://pubmed.ncbi.nlm.nih.gov/30343722/.
Cardiovascular Disease	African American patients are less likely than White patients to undergo diagnostic tests and revascularization, even after controlling for socioeconomic factors. Redberg, Rita F. "Gender, Race, and Cardiac Care." Journal of the American College of Cardiology 46, no. 10 (2005): 1852–54. https://doi.org/10.1016/j.jacc.2005.07.043. Gender, race, and Cardiac Care - jacc.org. Accessed February 5, 2024. https://www.jacc.org/doi/pdf/10.1016/j.jacc.2005.07.043.
Cardiovascular Disease	Black race significantly increases the risk of amputation, even within the same socioeconomic group compared with White patients and has an independent effect on limb loss after controlling for comorbidities, severity of PAD at presentation, and use of medications. Arya, Shipra, Zachary Binney, Anjali Khakharia, Luke P. Brewster, Phil Goodney, Rachel Patzer, Jason Hockenberry, and Peter W. Wilson. "Race and Socioeconomic Status Independently Affect Risk of Major Amputation in Peripheral Artery Disease." Journal of the American Heart Association 7, no. 2 (2018). https://doi.org/10.1161/jaha.117.007425. Arya, Shipra, Zachary Binney, Anjali Khakharia, Luke P. Brewster, Phil Goodney, Rachel Patzer, Jason Hockenberry, and Peter W. Wilson. "Race and Socioeconomic Status Independently Affect Risk of Major Amputation in Peripheral Artery Disease." Journal of the American Heart Association 7, no. 2 (January 23, 2018). https://doi.org/10.1161/jaha.117.007425.

Cerebrovascular Disease	African Americans are 50 percent more likely to have a stroke as compared to their White counterparts. Black men are 70 percent more likely to die from a stroke as compared to Whites. African American women are twice as likely to suffer from a stroke than White women. "Office of Minority Health." Home Page - Office of Minority Health (OMH). Accessed December 22, 2022. https://www.minorityhealth.hhs.gov/.
Infectious Diseases (HIV)	Disparities in the HIV care continuum persist in older age groups, particularly among African Americans. 　　Older African Americans face a disproportionate risk of acquiring HIV and suffer higher morbidity and mortality than older adults of other racial and ethnic groups. Sangaramoorthy, Thurka, Amelia Jamison, and Typhanye Dyer. "Older African Americans and the HIV Care Continuum: A Systematic Review of the Literature, 2003—2018." AIDS and Behavior 23, no. 4 (2018): 973—83. https://doi.org/10.1007/s10461-018-2354-4.
Renal Disease	African Americans over sixty-five years of age have death rates 15 percent greater than White. Hamler, Tyrone, Vivian Miller, and Sonya Petrakovitz. "Chronic Kidney Disease and Older African American Adults: How Embodiment Influences Self-Management." Geriatrics 3, no. 3 (2018): 52. https://doi.org/10.3390/geriatrics3030052.
Alzheimer's Disease	The age-related prevalence of dementia was 14 percent to100 percent higher in African Americans. The cumulative risk among first-degree relatives of African Americans who have Alzheimer's disease is 43.7 percent. There is a greater familial risk for Alzheimer's in African Americans. Genetic and environmental factors may work differently to cause Alzheimer's in African Americans "African Americans and Alzheimer's Disease: The Silent Epidemic." Alzheimer's Association. Accessed December 22, 2022. https://www.alz.org/media/seflorida/documents/afr amer.pdf. "New Alzheimer's Association Report Examines Racial and Ethnic Attitudes on Alzheimer's and Dementia." Alzheimer's Disease and Dementia. Accessed February 5, 2024. https://www.alz.org/news/2021/new-alzheimers-association-report-examines-racial.

Ocular Disease (Glaucoma)	Glaucoma-related blindness is between six and eight times more common among Black Americans than among White Americans. The authors studied population-based rates of incisional and laser surgery for open-angle glaucoma among Blacks and Whites in a 5 percent random sample of Medicare claims for 1986 through 1988. For all US Census divisions combined, the rate of surgery for glaucoma among Black beneficiaries was 2.2 times higher than the rate of surgery among White beneficiaries. The authors calculated an expected rate of glaucoma surgery was 45 percent lower than expected, which might in part account for the excess rate of blindness among Black Americans. The magnitude of the difference ranged from 29 percent in the Middle Atlantic states to 50 percent in the South Atlantic States. The authors concluded that African Americans are not receiving potentially sight-saving care for open-angle glaucoma at the same rate as White Americans. Javitt, Jonathan C., A. Marshall McBean, Geraldine A. Nicholson, J. Daniel Babish, Joan L. Warren, and Henry Krakauer. "Undertreatment of Glaucoma among Black Americans." New England Journal of Medicine 325, no. 20 (1991): 1418–22. https://doi.org/10.1056/nejm199111143252005.

Care Management Patient Information Tool (PIT)

THE PURPOSE OF THE TOOL:

Help educate the patient about their illness during hospitalization and post-hospitalization, increase the patient's knowledge base, create an environment where the patient is a collaborative partner while in the hospital and post-discharge, and most importantly, improve communication and understanding of the patient's concerns.

PIT is given to the patient upon admission by the care manager. It is not part of their medical record. A copy is given to the patient to continue to address concerns/questions with their primary care team or primary care doctor upon discharge. Patients used the tool to ask questions that may be forgotten while currently ill and fearful about their health outcome.

During Hospitalization
What am I being treated for? How long will I have this problem?
What other conditions/diagnoses do I have?

Ask your doctor or care team whether noncompliance or adherence, frequent flyer, etc. is written in your medical record.

Testing
What X-ray or test did I or will I have?
What was the result?

Medications
- I will be able to fill my prescriptions.
- I will not be able to fill my prescriptions.
- Is there a problem with taking herbal remedies along with my prescribed medications?
- How will my medication help me with my symptoms?
- Which medication helps which symptoms?
- How many do I take?
- How often should I take them?
- What side effects are important for me to call my doctor or hospital?

Family Involvement
When is a suitable time to talk with my family about my condition?

Medical Supplies—What Will I Need?
- Wound Dressing
- Oxygen
- Walker
- Other

Follow-Up Appointments
When is my follow-up appointment with my doctor?
I don't have a primary care doctor. Will I get one?
What is the doctor's name?

Diet
Do I need a special diet?

Homecare
Can I get homecare services to help me understand my medication and my condition?
Am I going home?
Am I going to a nursing home or rehab center?

My concerns while I am in the hospital:

1._____
2._____
3._____

When I Go Home . . .
What should I expect in terms of my symptoms when I go home?
Who should I call if I don't feel well before my doctor's appointment?

My concerns when I go home:
1._____
2._____

Recommended for discharge planning for nurses and social workers.

- Included should be a question about whether patients have a pill box.
- If the patient has a pill box, is it for morning, noon, and night or just for one time of day?
- If the patient does not have a pill box, should it be addressed prior to discharge planning?
- If homecare services will be provided, homecare nurses should set up the pill pox on the first visit to the patient's home

KCHC Medication Reconciliation Form for HOMECARE Agency

Patient Name
MR#
Discharge date
HC Agency name

1. ☐Yes ☐No
Are the discharge medications the same as the medications filled by the patient?
Comments

2. List all prescribed medications filled and dosage.
Comments

3. ☐Yes ☐No Are there additional prescribed medications in the home?
Comments

4. ☐Yes ☐No Are the medications in the home prescribed by a physician at KCHC or a community PCP?
Comments

5. If the medications were not prescribed by KCHC, indicate who the prescribing physician was and list the medications and physician contact information.
Comments

6. ☐Yes ☐No Are there herbal and or over-the-counter medicines?
If yes, list names of all medications.

7. ☐Yes ☐No Pillbox setup

8. ☐Yes ☐No Medication reconciliation completed

9. ☐Yes ☐No Medication reconciliation completed, and problems found:
Comment
10. Medication reconciliation incomplete or not done.

Reason

Signature:

NOTES

ACKNOWLEDGMENTS

I am eternally grateful to my medical training at Harlem Hospital, where excellent care was a mandate embedded in our brain under the leadership of Dr. Gerald Thomson. I would also like to recognize members of the Harlem Family who provided feedback on my book. Dr. Carolyn Britton, Dr. Denise Alveranga, Dr. Juan Bailey, Dr. Yves Jodesty, Dr. Brenda Bennett, Dr. Lawerence Brown, Dr. Al Ashford (R.I.P.) Dr. Don Dayson, Dr. Mary Bassett, and Dr. Dial Hewlett.

The Bridge Team: Sarah Lehernfeld, Associate Director Care Management, Prajakta Vagal, Director of Care Management, Marilyn McNair RN, Cynthia Cantos, Care Manager, Diana Hope, Social Worker.

Emergency Department Director, Dr. Stewart Kessler, Antonio Martin then CEO Kings County Hospital and the Congestive Heart Failure readmission team at Kings County—Dr. Reinaldo Austin, Dr. Augustine Umeozor, Pauline Hutchinson Case Manager, Wendy Gilles RN, Bolanle Bankole-Ogunlade RN, Assistant, Tamor Daley, Youselyn Champagne RN, Thamar Ferdinand Coordinating Manager, Miriam Klein, Pharmacist, Latoya Jackson RN, and Esther Bydeman, Social Worker.

Westchester Sickle Cell Outreach (WSCO), Kimberly Michelle Judon, BS, MPH, collaborative partner, and Dr. Danielle Nelson, Vice Chair, Department of Medicine. I also would like to acknowledge. Dr. Carol Bennett, Dr. Denise Jenkins, and Dr. Ernest Kendrick who, including myself, were 4-6 Blacks students who were pre-med at

Boston University and have supported each other along every step of the way, including providing key feedback about my book.

Equally important are the patients in our hospital beds that know who they are as individuals and that they are not just patients, and the stop-in-my-tracks moments that expanded my vision and improved the implementation processes.

Last, but not least, I would like to thank my amazing family: my husband Desmond Emanuel, my three sons Chase, Trent, and Ryan, my daughter in-law Alicia Emanuel, and my cousin Stephen McHayle for their unwavering support for my passion that led to me writing my book.

One thing that inspired me greatly was my mom's final statement before she met her maker. Two weeks prior to her passing, I visited my mother in the hospital to assess her cognitive function. I asked her, "Mom, who am I?"

Her response is forever embedded in my brain. She grabbed my hand and held it tightly and responded, "My dear, seek and you shall find."

Also thank you Mom and Dad for my Juneteenth Birthday. Rest in peace, Mom and Dad. I love you both and you are forever in my presence every day.

I would like to extend my appreciation to Dr. Irene Dankwa-Mullan, who provided key edits to my book. My appreciation to SteveHarrison, Co-Founder of The Bradley Communication Corporation and his team,Trish Ahjel Roberts, Christy Day, Cristina Smith, Valerie Costa, and Beth Volz. who worked to make my book shine.

My book pays homage to the individual patients of all races, ethnicities, and nationalities in our hospital beds and not in history books who were pivotal in inspiring the simple solutions woven throughout its pages.

CONTACT INFORMATION

How to Join My Community

If after reading this book you would like to get in touch with me, please visit my website at drbeverley.com.

You can also contact me at mbeverleymd@gmail.com.

Sign up for my mailing list
My blog/social media information

Speaking Engagement Information
To inquire about hiring me for speaking engagements, please contact me
at 914-409-2766 or mbeverleymd@gmail.com.

ABOUT THE AUTHOR

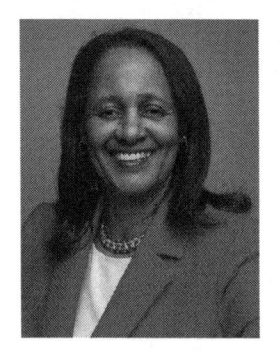

Mauvareen Beverley, M.D. is the President of Mauvareen Beverley, M.D., PLLC, Patient Engagement and Cultural Competence Specialist. She is an executive-level physician and a fellow of the New York Academy of Medicine (NYAM) with over twenty years of experience advocating for improving patient engagement and cultural competence for all populations, especially African American communities. As Assistant Vice President, Physician Advisor for NYC Health + Hospitals, she sponsored the first Conference on Improving the Health of the Elderly Black Population. Under her leadership as Deputy Executive Director of Kings County Hospital, she led her team to implement innovative strategies for improved equitable health outcomes and decreased Congestive Heart Failure readmission from 30 percent to 18.7 percent in less than two years.

Dr. Beverley is a national thought leader and expert in patient engagement and health equity. She has lectured extensively on health disparities, patient engagement and valuing the human experience. She collaborated with Westchester County Medical Society, Westchester Academy of Medicine, and Putnam County Medical Society in developing the Patient Engagement and Cultural Competence Training Program with CME credits and served as faculty of an education session for ACHE's Thomas C. Dolan Executive Diversity

Program. Her notable publications include "Patient Engagement and Cultural Sensitivity as a Strategy to Improve Health Inequities," which was published in the Journal of the National Medical Association. Her thought leadership paper on "Health Disparities and Epidemics: Perception vs. Reality" was selected for presentation at the New York Academy of Medicine's twelfth annual History of Medicine and Public Health Night in 2021. She received the Excellence in Medicine Award from the Bronx County Medical Society in 2021. She also made a scientific poster presentation on Solutions to Health Disparities: The Common Thread, The Human Experience presented at the American Hospital Association (AHA) Conference in Chicago, March 2022. Another poster, "Improving Health Disparities, The Common Thread: The Human Experience," was accepted to be displayed at the Institute of Healthcare Improvement (IHI) Forum December 13-15, 2022.

Dr. Beverley received her Bachelor of Science degree in biological sciences from Boston University and a medical degree from Jacob School of Medicine and Biomedical Science at the University of Buffalo School of Medicine. She trained in Internal Medicine at Harlem Hospital-NY Columbia Presbyterian. Dr. Beverley is a Member of The National Medical Association (NMA), The National Association of Health Service Executives (NAHSE), the American Medical Association (AMA), and the Medical Society, State of NY (MSSNY).